FOUNDATIONAL KNOWLEDGE For The PRACTICE OF FAMILY MEDICINE IN WEST AFRICA

FOUNDATIONAL KNOWLEDGE
For The
PRACTICE OF FAMILY MEDICINE IN WEST AFRICA

Victor Inem

Library of Congress Control Number:		2019906197
ISBN:	Hardcover	978-1-7960-3682-4
	Softcover	978-1-7960-3681-7
	eBook	978-1-7960-3680-0

Print information available on the last page.

Rev. date: 06/07/2019

To order additional copies of this book, contact:
Xlibris
1-888-795-4274
www.Xlibris.com
Orders@Xlibris.com
769089

CONTENTS

BOOK REVIEW

THE PARADIGM SHIFT from the original General medical practice to the current family medicine practice resulted in an obvious wide gap in knowledge and practice. It has been very imperative to write a book for fill this gap especially in the context of medical practice in West-African sub-region.

This book is a product of decades of practice, teaching and research in family medicine in Nigeria and other countries in Africa and beyond. It set out to update the missing link between practitioners of family medicine in the tropics and to provide the foundational basis of family medicine to upcoming practitioners in the field.

The book brings together the basic foundation principles, concepts and theories upon which the practice of family medicine is built.

It addresses the family medicine concept of what a family is, and with special emphasis on the different family models used in the assessment and evaluation of individual and family health status.

It clearly elucidates the basis and concept of systems thinking, biopsycho-social theory and various assessment tools used in family medicine diagnosis and management. The roles and responsibilities of a family physician are clearly highlighted. The challenges of managing the myriads of undifferentiated health conditions and uncertainties of illness in family practice are highlighted.

The role of family functionality and social support in the prevention of disease and promotion / maintenance of health was clearly articulated.

The applications of all these principles and concepts to the practice and training of family physicians in Africa, makes this book a must read for all family physicians practicing in the West African sub-region.

Dr. ShabiOlabode
Chief Consultant Family Physician
Federal Teaching Hospital
Ado-Ekiti
Ekiti State

Senior Lecturer
Afe Babalola University
Ado-Ekiti

Editor,
Nigerian Journal of Family Practice.

ACKNOWLEDGEMENT

MOST IMPORTANTLY FOR me is my gratitude to God Almighty for this dream which has been embryonic for more than 12 years come through.

I also thank my numerous colleagues and friends especially Dr. O. A. Ewedairo who contributed the chapter on Family Support and Dr. T. E. Attoye who took time to edit the entire manuscript. Incidentally both were my residents who went on to receive postgraduate training at the prestigious Harvard University. They believed so much in me and took me on as their mentor. My Personal Assistant Mr. Olawale Oladejo, Ph.D. Medical Physics (in view) who accommodated my idiosyncrasies and Ms Joy Daniels for secretarial assistance and many others who God used to complete this work.

Finally, I appreciate God's invaluable gift to me, Grace Cobham Inem and my children. TO GOD BE THE GLORY.

DEDICATION

THIS WORK IS dedicated to my highly cherished parents His Serene Highness Etidung Elder Victor Inem of blessed memory and my mum, the Queen mother, Eka, my family friends the Alonges, Ogundes, Okojies and Akpan families who contributed immensely to my early education and developmental upbringing. Though some are long gone to be with the Lord their efforts were not in vain. Glory to God.

PREFACE

THIS BOOK IS written for medical students, resident doctors of the National Postgraduate Medical Ccollege and the West African College of Physicians in the faculty of Family medicine as well as those reading for the diploma in family medicine.

The first medical degree MBBS or MBChB is the primordial step or the stem cell to practice. This does not in any way confer the status of General Practitioner to a medical graduate. To practice as a GP even with this first degree requires continuing professional development. For this reason a Doctor needs to be trained in General Practice which is a narrow but essential part that forms the more comprehensive and larger specialty of Family Medicine.

Family Medicine is a distinct discipline with its own science cum art form and not a subspecialty of any other discipline. Family Medicine is firmly entrenched in Primary and Secondary care with subspecialty in the areas of lifestyle medicine, emergency care, geriatric and palliative care among others.

The "foundational knowledge" is needed as the baseline on which family medicine practice stands. Once the basics are gotten right, the understanding and application of the concepts are made a lot easier. However, when the very beginning which is the base is weak or faulty, conceptualization and contextualization of necessary principles and processes of the subject becomes difficult and the application wrong. Invariably, this leads to frustration and loss of interest in the specialty.

Two principal reasons motivated the writing of this book. First I met one of my former students, a Diplomate in Family Medicine and Professor of Rural Surgery who had practiced in diverse places like Saudi Arabia, England and rural Nigeria and who felt that the absence of written texts concerning the unique features of the specialty especially in the West African context was like winking in the dark. He also felt that the inadequate focus on the need for doctors to be trained in Family Medicine was a big disservice to both the medical and non-medical West African communities.

Secondly, a colleague in a more familiar specialty once asked me – as many others have since asked, "What are you teaching that has not been taught by the other specialists?" I informed him that there is more breadth than depth in family medicine in the synthesis of the generalist context in a specialist mode, an understanding of the oxymoronic nature of the specialty. The basic science on which Family Medicine is founded includes the details on various subjects concerning the family in the area of social sciences of sociology psychology anthropologic concepts that has guided this foundational knowledge. These thoughts culminated in the idea of writing down, however briefly, an explanation of what we practice.

I have therefore been challenged to write this book in which I have described the various steps taken to bring the faculty to fruition. This book provides a comprehensive base in a readable and friendly format. The 10 chapters are related in many ways and have several areas of overlap that have necessitated their being put together.

This book is not in any way exhaustive of the subjects, but it highlights the essentials of the subjects that form the foundation of family medicine. Therefore, students, teachers as well as researchers who desire to grasp the foundation in family medicine for research and practice will find this book an appropriate companion.

It is in this respect that this book will satisfy the needs of its users because it bridges the gap between the mish-mash of biomedical with social sciences as the basic sciences of family medicine and the clinical skills needed to practice in this environment.

Prof. Victor Inem

CHAPTER 1

What Is a Family?

THE FAMILY IS so significant to humanity that it is universal – every human group in the world organizes its members in families. It is the interface of the individual with the larger society. It is the smallest social group. Friedman says that the family "forms the basic unit of our society and so strongly influences development of an individual that it may determine the success or failure of that person's life". The family unit occupies a position between the individual and society.

There are many definitions of the family. In the typical Western societies, the nuclear family comprises of a married couple and their children by birth or adoption.

This limiting definition implies those who are legally married and their children. This definition is no longer sufficient because of trends towards independence and alternative lifestyle. Today this nuclear family does not represent the majority of families in West Africa. A composition and structural definition would include kinship members with differentiated positions in a family system, such as grandparents, uncles, nieces, aunts and any other genetic relatives. Functionally a family is any group engaged in certain family activities such as child rearing, nurturing socialization etc. The family can also be defined as a group of 2 or more people living together who are committed to each other. These people may be or may not be related by marriage or genetics but they care about each other. This definition encompasses a much more diverse group.

In today's society, the family is the basic biological, psychological, and sociological unit. Sometimes legal implications are also considered important in looking at a family. As a *biological* unit, the family produces children, who may inherit genetic traits or have a predisposition to specific health problems such as depression, diabetes, or heart disease. The family as a *psychological* unit interacts with members of the nuclear family and often extended family members, such as grandparents, step-parents, aunts, uncles, and cousins. Family relationships and interactions may profoundly influence each member's values, beliefs, and behaviors.

Sociological aspects of the family include the multiple role and activities or tasks that members carry out both within the family structure and in the community. Ethnic and cultural values, traditions, and practices are often passed on and guide younger family members' behavior patterns. Roles and activities may be viewed within the context of working, learning, socializing, child-rearing, house-keeping, exercising, community functioning, religion, and so forth.

The *legal* aspects of the family are found in definitions of the state and local laws, which may impact on the family. For example, decisions regarding who qualifies to pay child support and who is considered a "family member" with visitation privileges in a hospital are determined by legal interpretations.

Definition of a Family

Anthropologists have pointed out that the definition of what constitutes a family is not universal. The world's cultures display so much variety that the term *family* is difficult to define. For instance, if we were to define the family as the unit in which parents are responsible for disciplining children and providing for their material needs, this would not be a universal definition.

As a case in point, among the Trobri and Islanders, it is not the parents but the wife's eldest brother who is responsible for providing the children's discipline and their food.

Such remarkable variety requires a broad and encompassing definition. Definitions differ depending on theoretical orientation of the definer i.e. biological, sociological, psychological, legal, political etc.

"Two or more persons who are joined together by bonds of sharing and emotional closeness and who identify themselves as being part of the family."

In light of the biological, psychological, and sociological implications of the Family on a patient, the discipline of Family medicine therefore focuses on the patient in the context of the family. For our purposes, families are defined in the context of the index patient i.e. they decide who they consider family and we accept the following as a definition of the Family;

> *The Family is defined as a social and intimate nurturing group of individuals connected to a patient biologically, legally, or by choice, from whom the patient can reasonably expect a measure of support in the form of food, shelter, finance and emotional nurturing; that share a past, a present and a future with the patient and includes all who contribute in one way or the other to the family culture.*

A **family** therefore consists of people who consider themselves related by blood, marriage, or adoption. The concept of a **household** is a related but distinct demographic construct which consists of people who occupy the same housing unit – a house, apartment, or other living quarters. In demographic terms in West Africa – a group of people eating from the same pot.

The concept of a family as an entity is an abstraction whose reality varies from place to place. There is wide cross-cultural variation in patterns of kinship, with many different types of family structure.

CLASSIFICATION OF FAMILIES:

Sociologists refer to the **family of orientation** (the family in which an individual grows up) and the **family of procreation** (the family that is formed when a couple have their first child). Broadly speaking, we can classify families as **nuclear** (husband, wife, and children) and **extended** (including people such as grandparents, aunts, uncles, and cousins in addition to the nuclear unit) with some variations within each group.

a. Nuclear family consists of a father, a mother and their children. Variations:

    i. The blended or step parent family also called the reconstituted family. (each divorced parent brings their children into the new union)

    ii. The "Binuclear" family: a divorced couple with joint custody of the children.

    iii. The Single parent family: One-parent with children; usually mother-children.

    iv. The Nuclear dyad family: a couple with no children.

    v. Single adult living alone.

    1. Homosexual Gay/lesbian families: This is an area where legal definition of family has become increasingly important. Essentially the same as a nuclear family but couple is of same sex.

b. Polygamous families: In this type of family, men have more than one wife (**polygyny**) or women more than one husband (**polyandry**). It has been practiced in many cultures, most commonly men having several wives.

c. Extended family: nuclear family plus other relatives, usually multi-generational, may live in the same household or a number or households, usually near each other.

d. Communal families group of people living together, consider themselves families, share work, responsibilities and property to varying degrees. The commitment to relationships is also variable.

e. Skip-generation families: In which a child is being raised grandparents.
f. Joint family: a household composed of married siblings' spouses and children
g. On a larger scale, a group of people may define themselves as a family based on descendant from a common ancestor several generations in the past.

SOME FUNCTIONS OF THE FAMILY

- Pass on culture (e.g., religion, ethnicity)
- Socialize young people for the next generation
- Exist for sexual satisfaction and reproduction
- Provide economic security
- Serve as a protective mechanism for family members against outside forces
- Provide closer human contact and relations
- Physical maintenance and health care

LEVELS OF INTERACTION WITH THE FAMILY IN FAMILY MEDICINE

This relates to how or who we view as the client/patient as well as the type of care provided

a. The Client as an identified individual (like your patient in the hospital). The interactions with his/her family are the larger context in which the client may be viewed.
b. The Client as the family as a whole. Here the whole family is systematically assessed. Interventions are aimed at family system, and how it relates to larger systems.
c. The Family as a component of society either in research or therapy, for example with dysfunctional families, families would be referred to them by GPs or other specialist working at the other 2 level the identified individual/holistic view.

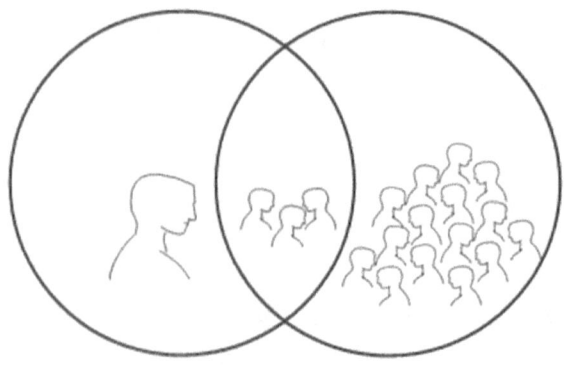

Family:- Interface of Individual with the society

CHAPTER 2

SYSTEMS THINKING IN FAMILY MEDICINE

T HINKING IN TERMS of systems rather than isolated parts is crucial to the practice of family medicine. A system is defined as a whole, made of interactive parts. The interaction between these components result in a whole that is greater than the sum of its component parts. A *system* consists of a set of interacting components within a boundary that filters the type and rate of exchange with the environment. Systems are composed of both structural and functional components. Structure refers to the arrangements of the parts at a given time; function is the process of continuous change in the system as matter, energy, and information are exchanged with the environment.

All living systems are *open* in that there is continual exchange of matter, energy, and information. In open systems there are varying degrees of interaction with the environment from which the system receives input and gives back output in the form of matter, energy, and information. Theoretically, no closed systems exist, as they would be totally isolated from interaction with the environment.

The universe consists of a *hierarchy* of systems (numerous suprasystems, systems, and subsystems), and each system may be viewed as having one or more suprasystems and subsystems. For example, the individual as a system belongs to suprasystems in a family, community, and region. An individual's subsystems are composed of organ systems or biopsychosocial components.

Each system has discrete, definable boundaries that filter and regulate the flow of input and output exchange with the environment. Boundaries may consist of physical or abstract lines of demarcation that separate the system from the surrounding environment. The filter may be very impermeable, or fairly impermeable, depending on the component it is screening in or out of the system.

For survival, all systems must receive varying types and amounts of matter, energy, and information from the environment. Through the process of selection, the system regulates the type and amount of *input* received.

A system must continuously monitor itself and the environment for information to guide its operations. This *feedback* information of environmental responses to the system's output is utilized by the system in adjustment, correction, and accommodation to the interaction with the environment. Feedback may be positive, negative, or neutral.

For survival, a system must achieve a balance internally and externally. *Equilibrium* depends on the ability of the system to regulate input and output with the environment to achieve a balanced relationship of the interacting parts. Because balance is continually changing, a self-regulating mechanism within the system monitors the interaction of inputs and outputs with the environment by using information from feedback. Through interactions with the environment, the system uses various *adaptation* mechanisms to maintain equilibrium. Adaptation may occur through accepting or rejecting the matter, energy, or information and by accommodating the input and modifying the system's responses to maintain or regain equilibrium.

SYSTEMS THEORY

General systems theory serves as a model for viewing man as interacting with the environment. One of the first theorists to develop systems theory was Ludwig von Bartalanffy (1968), who synthesized the following abstract laws in systems theory development:

1. Systems are organized complexities in which behavior is determined by interaction among various components.

2. No system repeats its interaction, but continuous interaction among variables produces uniquely dynamic situations infinitely.
3. Evolution proceeds from a less to a more differentiated state; dynamic interaction between individuals and the environment results in increasing complexity for both.
4. Regular changes are found in the evolution of all systems as they move toward higher states of order, differentiation, and probability.
5. People are living, open, metabolizing systems, exhibiting self-differentiation, providing energy, and having a stored information system (genetic code) to steer the process.

GENERAL SYSTEMS THEORY (GST) IN FAMILY MEDICINE

Most clinicians trained after 1980 would have encountered general systems theory in one form or the other during the study of physiology and it argues that such seemingly non-mathematical and imprecise concepts as "health", "medical care" can be better understood by applying the GST. George Engel melded the GST with his biopsychosocial model of medicine for the purpose of more comprehensively viewing the medical care of the person and tailored the application of GST to the family being part of the person's biological and social systems hierarchy. The point has sometimes been made that a biological entity, such as a person or community, is far too complex to be viewed in such a seemingly rigid fashion, that the world is a random and swirling milieu or ethereal entities and ill-defined forces. Therefore a flexible approach has to be taken in the use of this theory. The System theory is applicable in the family medicine process of the individual, family, and community client. It is frequently used to assess and analyze a community.

GENERAL SYSTEMS THEORY AND THE HIERARCHY OF SYSTEM

The application of GST to any biological system involves three principles;

1. All natural entities and phenomena can be organized into specific systems that share properties.
2. These systems can then be organized into a hierarchy such that each system contains certain subsystems and is itself a subsystem.
3. The forces impacting both positively and negatively, on any particular system can also be viewed in a generic way, both as to origin and effect.

Each level in the hierarchy is self-contained but interdependent upon the levels above (supra-systems) and blow (sub-systems). The level influences each other via feedback loops. This hierarchy represents all of its component levels in an ultimate fashion because it serves not only to define the boundaries (e. g., of persons composed of organs composed of tissue composed of cell, etc.), or family composed of individual, community composed of families etc. but also to provide the structure (organization in space) upon which forces important to each level may be projected.

THE PERSON AND THE FAMILY IN GENERAL SYSTEMS THEORY

The General Systems Theory helps to clarify the intimate, yet confusing relationship between the family and its members. References to the family as the unit of medical care usually mean medical care directed towards the individual in the context of the family, including vectors of infectious disease, stress-related illness, provision of logistical and/or emotional support, effects on treatment compliance, or availability of rehabilitative support.

Actually, the family is an entity in its own right, is capable of experiencing distress, dysfunction, disruption and discoordination in role definition. It is the incorporation of these types of "family disease" into the West African Medical care model (conflicts at individual level-gender violence, harmful traditional practices and corporate conflicts like communal conflict, wars, refugees, human right violations, disasters) that require attention by family physicians if medical care is to be actually applied to the family as a unit.

Laszlo, Brody and Antonovsky defined 'health' as the harmonious interaction of all systems in the hierarchy containing person and family. Conversely, 'disease' is defined as non-accommodated perturbations (disturbance) in the hierarchy that cause disharmony. In disease, some adverse force impacts at one or more levels; this is known as the 'initial perturbation'. In theoretical terms, at least, that force is felt throughout the hierarchy as a result of subsequent 'accommodation disruptions', although these may be imperceptible at certain levels. The resulting disruption may spread with a ripple effect.

The origin of most conflict emanates from the ability or inability at the family level to resolve these so-call non-medical issues or "family disease" that eventually spirals into the clinic, emergency room or wards as trauma, malnutrition, health promotive and rehabilitative encounter etc. with the family physicians.

The family can generate its own internal support as a protective mechanism, as well as obtain support from other natural systems in its own hierarchy or in other hierarchies. Any natural system in the hierarchy can be the source of both noxious and supportive forces, with the more adjacent levels of Person and Community being relatively more important as a source of both.

However, the internal support systems of a family are likely more important as a dampening and modifying influence on the initial perturbations and accommodation disruptions described previously.

The type of forces is provided by Smilkstein and summarized by his acronym SCREEM, grouped into; six types of forces, namely **Social**: including factors such as medical care, leisure time resources, and community networks and organizations that impact most immediately on the patient, **Cultural**; including religious factors which are closely related to ethnic and racial background. **Economic**: including level of **Education** and type and level of **Employment**, all three 'Es' being closely intertwined. **Medico-Political:** including legal and policy decisions, usually originating at the national level.

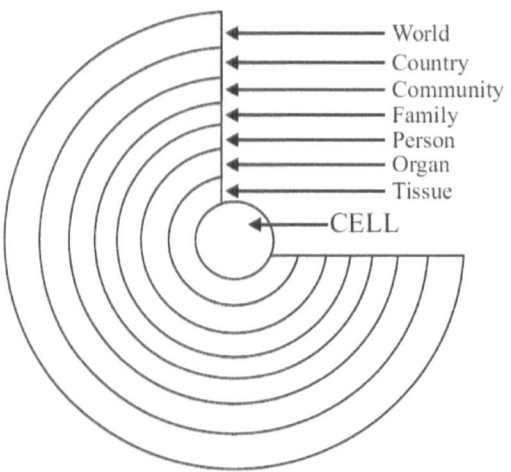

FAMILY SYSTEMS

A family system is a social or biological construct made up of a set of people related by blood or intention. Members interact in reciprocal relationships responding to one another in this context.

HOW FAMILY SYSTEM OPERATES

Each family describes and defines for itself the way their family system will operate. Each family type therefore can be thought of as a separate family culture, which has underlying group norms, roles, behaviors and expectations. The nature of this culture depends on the following:

a. **That Families are Interactive** – i.e. there is the interplay between members.
b. **That the parties within the family reciprocate** – both parties influence each other as they interact (interplay between members) with each other.
c. **That there are roles** – a character or function one plays.

CHARACTERISTICS OF THE FAMILY SYSTEM

FAMILY COMMUNICATION

Communication within the family system could be verbal or nonverbal and it includes rules within the system. Communication could range from good or bad and this affects the overall functioning of the system.

CHANGE AND STABILITY

Family systems are stable in their chaos and orderly in their disorder. Families are predictable in general and unpredictable in detail, thus the need to study each individually.

HOMEOSTASIS

This is the ability of a system to return to a state of equilibrium, this is counteracted in the need for change in a long system.

SUBSYSTEM

These are smaller units inside the layer system that share the characteristics of the larger system and could have multiple identities within the larger family system.

FEEDBACK LOOPS

This is the "part along which information can be traced from one point in a system, through one or more parts of the systems or its environment and back to the point of origin.

Feedback loops are of two types, positive and negative. A negative feedback loop has been linked to the homeostasis system, in which the feedback loop provides information that returns to some present level and reduce deviation to a system while the positive feedback loop tends to promote or provide change.

TASKS FOR THE FAMILY PHYSICIAN IN APPLYING FAMILY SYSTEMS TO PRACTICE

Family mapping
Family Characteristic – members
Family Structure – boundaries, alliances, coalitions
Family Processes – enhancement, disengagement.
Family Accreting – intergeneration, coalitions

CHAPTER 3

GENERAL MODELS

MASLOW'S HIERARCHY OF NEEDS

ADVOCATES OF HUMAN needs theory view individuals as integrated, whole beings who are motivated by internal and external needs that create tension. To reduce this tension, an individual seeks to meet specific needs through goal-directed behavior. Abraham Maslow classified human needs into five categories of predominance and placed them in a hierarchy. This hierarchy of human needs begins with basic fundamental needs of the individual that must be satisfied before proceeding to the next higher level. Throughout life the individual strives to satisfy needs at each level, but at different periods need within one or more categories may be predominant. The desire to gratify human needs at each level motivates the individual and strengthens goal-directed behaviors. Generally, basic physiological needs and safety needs must be relatively satisfied in the individual before he or she can strive for higher level needs.

BASIC NEEDS

Physiological needs are the physical requirements for human survival. If these requirements are not met, the human body cannot function properly and will ultimately fail. Physiological needs are thought to be the most important; they should be met first.

A variety of fundamental physical needs have been identified, including air, food, sleep, sex, fluids, exercise, elimination, and stimulation. For survival and satisfactory functioning, every individual must have these basic physiological needs met. The extent or degree to which each of these needs is met varies with the individual. Some people require more sleep or food than others, but individuals must satisfy these needs at their own specific levels.

SAFETY

When basic physical needs are relatively satisfied, safety needs emerge; these include security, stability, order, physical safety, freedom from fear, protection, and sometimes dependency. These needs reflect self-protection through the establishment of structure, law, order, and limits.

Needs for safety and protection from harm may become more prominent when the individual is threatened by bodily harm, as in physical illness or potential injury. Safety needs involve both imminent danger or concerns and potential loss, such as loss of the security of a spouse or an occupational position.

With their physical needs relatively satisfied, the individual's safety needs take precedence and dominate behavior. In the absence of physical safety – due to war, natural disaster, family violence, childhood abuse, etc. – people may (re-)experience post-traumatic stress disorder or transgenerational trauma. In the absence of economic safety – due to economic crisis and lack of work opportunities – these safety needs manifest themselves in ways such as a preference for job security, grievance procedures for protecting the individual from unilateral authority, savings accounts, insurance policies, reasonable disability accommodations, etc. This level is more likely to be found in children because they generally have a greater need to feel safe.

Safety and Security needs include:

- *Personal security*
- *Financial security*
- *Health and well-being*
- *Safety net against accidents/illness and their adverse impacts*

SELF FULFILMENT NEED

When the lower needs in the hierarchy have been relatively satisfied, an individual strives towards self-actualization. Young people may grow toward self-actualization, but must usually reach maturity before they have a sense of self-actualization. Self-actualization means that the individual is relatively satisfied with most aspects of life. This includes what the person thinks of self and the level of achievement reached or the ability to fulfill that designated purpose in life. Some adults continue working toward self-actualization all their lives; others arrive at a sense of fulfillment or accomplishment in mid-life. The individual feels a sense of having achieved a purpose in life and having developed capabilities to fullest.

SELF-ACTUALIZATION

What a man can be, he must be." This quotation forms the basis of the perceived need for self-actualization. This level of need refers to what a person's full potential is and the realization of that potential. Maslow describes this level as the desire to accomplish everything that one can, to become the most that one can be. Individuals may perceive or focus on this need very specifically. For example, one individual may have the strong desire to become an ideal parent. In another, the desire may be expressed athletically. For others, it may be expressed in paintings, pictures, or inventions. As previously mentioned, Maslow believed that to understand this level of need, the person must not only achieve the previous needs, but master them.

SELF-TRANSCENDENCE

In his later years, Maslow explored a further dimension of needs, while criticizing his own vision on self-actualization. The self only finds its actualization in giving itself to some higher goal outside oneself, in altruism and spirituality is emphasized in family member care.

Maslow's hierarchy of needs is a broad model. The deficiency of basic needs are said to motivate people when they are unmet. Also, the need to fulfil such needs will become stronger the longer the duration they are denied. For example, the longer a person goes without food the more hungry they will become.

One must satisfy lower level basic needs before progressing on to meet higher level growth needs. Once these needs have been reasonably satisfied, one may be able to reach the highest level called self-actualization.

Every person is capable and has the desire to move up the hierarchy toward a level of self-actualization. Unfortunately, progress is often disrupted by failure to meet lower level needs. Life experiences, including divorce and loss of job may cause an individual to fluctuate between levels of the hierarchy.

Maslow noted only one in a hundred people become fully self-actualized because our society rewards motivation primarily based on esteem, love and other social needs. It is applicable to individual and family clients. Although the family physicians can assist clients to meet the first four needs, the fifth need, self-actualization, is generally left to the client to meet after other needs are met.

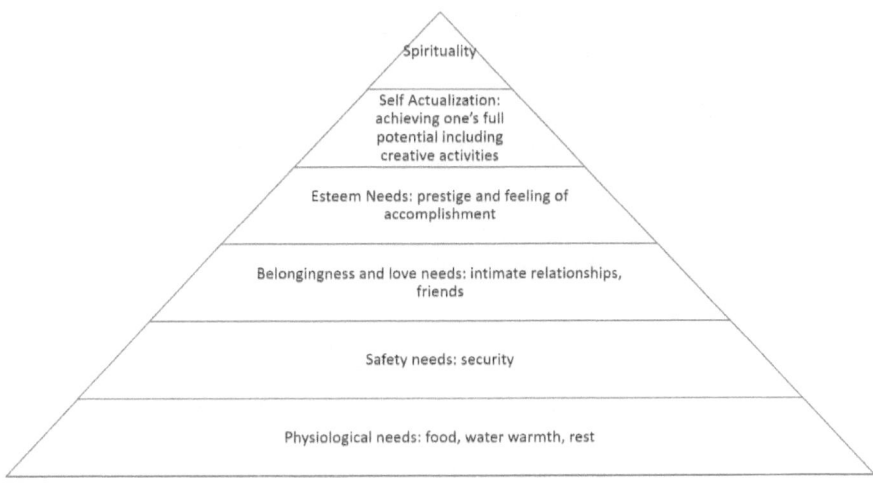

JOHARI WINDOW

The Johari Window is a communication model that is used to improve understanding between individuals. The word "Johari" is taken from the names of Joseph Luft and Harry Ingham, who developed the model in 1955.

There are two key ideas behind the tool:

1. That you can build trust with others by disclosing information about yourself.
2. That, with the help of feedback from others, you can learn about yourself and come to terms with personal issues.

By explaining the idea of the Johari Window, you can help team members to understand the value of self-disclosure, and you can encourage them to give, and accept, constructive feedback. Done sensitively, this can help people build better, more trusting relationships with one another, solve issues, and work more effectively as a team.

The family Physician – Patient dyad is conserved to restore health, prevent disease and rehabilitation.

1 Known Self Things we know about ourselves and others know about us	2 Hidden Self Things we know about ourselves that others do not know
3 Blind Self Things others know about us that we do not know	4 Unknown Self Things neither we nor others know about us

Fig 3: Johari Window Theory X and Y

CHAPTER 4

FAMILY MODELS

THE USE OF a specific family model provides a perspective or focus for understanding the family. Family models have been categorized according to their basic focus as developmental, interactional, structural-functional, and system models. First, two family developmental models, Duvall's and Stevenson's are presented. Next, Satir's family interactional model is described. Friedman's structural-focus, as does Calgary' family model, which also includes the system approach. There are many other family models available.

DUVALL'S FAMILY DEVELOPMENTAL MODEL

Evelyn Duvall's (1977) family developmental framework provides a guide to examine and analyze the basic changes and developmental tasks common to most families during their life cycle. Although each family has characteristics, normative patterns of sequential developmental tasks (see Table 4-1) illustrate common family behaviors that may be expected at specific times in the family life cycle. The stages of family development are marked by the age of the oldest child, although there is some overlapping of stages when there are several children in the family.

Stage I (*beginning families*) begins with the married couple as they establish a mutually satisfying relationship. The couple's tasks center on forming an intimate relationship and balance in their lives together, family planning, and establishing a harmonious relationship with in-laws and new friends. Adjusting to pregnancy and planning for parenthood are also critical tasks during this stage.

Stage II (*early childbearing*) begins when the first child between birth and 30 months; at this time the family tasks involve adjusting to the critical needs and demands of an infant while continuing to establish a satisfying home environment. Changes in roles and responsibilities with parenthood are critical tasks.

Table 4-1: Duvall's Family Developmental Stages and Tasks

Stages of Development The Basic family tasks

Stages of Development	The Basic family tasks
i. Beginning families	1. Physical maintenance
ii. Early childbearing	2. Allocation of resources
iii. Families with preschooler	3. Division of labor
iv. Families with school children	4. Socialization of members
v. Families with teenagers	5. Reproduction, recruitment, and release of members
vi. Launching center families	6. Maintenance of order
vii. Middle-aged families	7. Placement of member in the larger society
viii. Aging families	8. Maintenance of motivation and moral

Stage III (*families with preschooler*) begins as the parent adapt to the challenging needs and interests of the preschool child in a way to promote the child's growth. In adapting to the preschooler's needs, the parent may find their energy and privacy reduced. With the addition of another infant, parent may experience increased child-rearing responsibilities and the need for more living space in the home and more personal time to maintain intimacy and communication.

Stage IV (*families with school children*) begins as the oldest child enters school; the family tasks revolve around adjusting to community activities involving the child, encouraging the child's educational achievement, and maintaining a satisfying marital relationship. Critical tasks include balancing time and energy to meet the demands of work, the children's needs and activities, adult social interests, and the requirements of open communication and harmony in the marital and in-law relationship.

Stage V (*families with teenager*) begin when the oldest child become a teenager; a gradual emancipation commences as the child develop increasing independence and autonomy. Families with teenager must adapt to balancing freedom for growth with meeting family responsibilities. Critical tasks during this period are maintaining open communication between parent and teenager, continuing intimacy in the marital relationship, and establishing outside interest and careers as teenagers leave the home.

Stage VI (*launching center families*) begins when the first child has left. Parents must both prepare their children to live independently and accept the departure of the children. After the children have left, the parent must reorganize to reestablish the family unit. Husband and wife roles and responsibilities will shift during this period if the wife returns to work. With the birth of grandchildren, parental roles and self-images require some family accommodation.

Stage VII (*middle-aged families*) begins after the children have left the home, when middle-aged parent have more time and freedom to cultivate their social and leisure interests. This may also be a period for rebuilding the marriage and maintaining satisfying relationship both with aging parent and with the children and their families. Planning for retirement while maintaining physical and emotional health and careers are major family concerns.

Stage VIII (*aging families*) begins with retirement of one or both spouses and continues until the deaths of both marital partners. Critical tasks focus on finding sufficient energy and motivation to seek and engage in pleasurable leisure activities within financial and health limitations. Major tasks are adjusting to retirement with changing lifestyles and accepting the deaths of friends and spouse. Within this period the family may also close the home and move into a retirement community, thus having to establish ties with new friends in a new community and to find new leisure activities.

Within each of the successive stages of family development, Duvall identified eight basic tasks, as shown in Table 1-1, that lead to successful family life within society. These tasks promote family adjustment and adaptation of the individual members. When families fail to accomplish these tasks, the family collectively or its members individually may experience unhappiness, societal disapproval, and difficulty in achieving harmony and self-actualization. The family tasks involve responsibilities to satisfy the biological, cultural, and personal needs and aspirations of the members at each stage of family development.

These eight basic tasks include the following:

1. *Physical maintenance*: The family is responsible for providing shelter, appropriate clothing, sufficient nourishing food, and adequate health care.
2. *Allocation of resources:* these resources include finances, personal time, energy, and relationship. Family members' needs are met through division of cost and labor to provide material goods, space, and facilities, and through interpersonal relations to share authority, respect, and affection.
3. *Division of labor.* Family members decide who will assume what responsibilities, such as providing income, managing the house

hold tasks, maintaining the home and car, caring for young, old, or incapacitated family members, and other designated tasks.

4. *Socialization of family members*: The family assumes responsibilities for guiding development of mature and acceptable patterns of socially acceptable behavior in eating, elimination, sleeping, sexually, aggression, and interaction with others.

5. *Reproduction, recruitment, and release of family members*: Childbearing, adoption, and rearing of children are family responsibilities, along with incorporating new members through marriage. Policies are established for including others in the family, such as in-laws relatives, step-parents, guests, and friends.

6. *Maintenance of order*: Order is maintained by the communication of acceptable behavior. The types of intensity of interactions, patterns of affection, and sexual expression are sanctioned by parental behavior to ensure acceptance in society.

7. *Placement of members in the larger society*: Family members establish roots in society through relationship in the church, school, political and economic system, and other organizations. The family also assumes responsibility for protecting family members from undesirable outside influences and may prohibit membership in objectionable groups.

8. *Maintenance of motivation and morale*: Family members reward each other for their achievement and provide for an individual's needs of acceptances, encouragement, and affection. The family develops philosophy of life and sense of family unity and loyalty, thereby enabling members to adapt to both personal and family crises.

Duvall's developmental model is an excellent guide for assessing, analyzing, and planning around basic family tasks at a specific developmental stage. However, this model does not include the family structure or physiological aspects, which should be considered for a comprehensive view of the family. The model is applicable for nuclear families with growing children, and families who are experiencing health-related problems.

SATIR'S INTERACTIONAL FAMILY MODEL

Virginia Satir (1972) believes that the family's interactional health depends on its ability to share and understand the members' feelings, needs, and behavior patterns. She thinks that healthy, nurturing families help their members know themselves through communication n of everyday events. This communication promotes each individual's self-confidence and self-worth. Satir views the healthy family as hopeful, trusting of other, and curious about what society has to offer. The family operates on a growth-producing, reality-oriented basis. This promotes intimacy among its members. Family rules about money, chores, and power are explicit and understood by everyone. Also, the healthy family establishes links with society. These links are established through membership in various groups. Satir's model of the healthy family consists of four concepts: **self-worth, communication, rules, and links to the society**. Family members and family units demonstrate feeling of high esteem and self-worth. These attitudes are conveyed by behaviors showing integrity, honesty, responsibility, compassion, and love. These attitudes flow outward from each individual, and a sense of trust radiates from all members. They accept their own strengths and inadequacies as well as those of others. Without self-worth, family members build walls of distrust, isolation, and loneliness. They fear others will cheat them, use them, or step on them. This leads to unhealthy family interaction.

Communication directly influences the relationship among family members. Patterns of communication include body movement, posture, tone of voice, and spoken words. In healthy families, communication is open, direct, clear, and honest. The members are receptive and encourage open, honest sharing of feelings and needs. They value what others have to say, supporting each member's attempts in both verbal and physical communication. Unhealthy families block communication among members; they may give ambiguous messages or not listen at all. This leads to distrust and low self-worth among the family members.

Each family has a set of rules it lives by. These rules may be explicit or implicit. Most families assume that everyone knows and understands the rules, but this is not always true. Families have rules about money, responsibilities, activities, special privileges, privacy, sexual expression, language, territoriality, and authority. In many situations, rules define what actions are appropriate; they may also guide how feelings are expressed and may help achieve goals or impede goal achievement. Some rules may be outdated, unfair, unclear, or inappropriate. In healthy families the rules are known to all members, allow for freedom, and encourage discussion among the members.

Unhealthy families may have implicit rules that restrict family members. These rules may be inflexible and inhabit the growth of the members.

The family unit and individual members have *links to society* through organization and friends. The organizational links include school, church, political groups, recreational group, and clubs. Links with friends are usually formed through common interests. With these links the family and its members keep actively involved in the community and relate to the world around them. Healthy families have many links with society, believing society has much to offer and trusting their selection of groups to be a positive influence and interaction. They believe society offers opportunities for choices and changed, growth, and developmental. These opportunities are welcomed, desirable, and normal. Unhealthy families views society with distrust and fear exposure to other's values. They avoid involvement in organization, preferring to remain isolated. They do not welcome experiences outside the family.

Satir's interactional family model addresses four major psychosocial concept considered important in a healthy family. The model is limited because it does not include family structure, function, and developmental level. The model can be applied to any type of family, but additional model may be necessary.

FRIEDMAN'S STRUCTURAL-FUNCTIONAL FAMILY MODEL

Friedman's family model was developed from sociological frameworks and system theory by Marilyn Friedman (1986). The family is focus of the model, as it interacts with suprasystems in the community and with individual family members in the subsystem. The model is comprised of two components – structural and functional – as shown in Table 4-2. The structural component examines the family unit, how it is organized, and how members relate to one another in terms of their values, communication network, role systems, and power. The functional component refers to the interactional outcomes resulting from the family organizational structure. The structural-functional component and part all intimately interrelate and interact: each component and part is affected by the others.

CHAPTER 5

BIOPSYCHOSOCIAL CONCEPTS

ONE OF THE most widely accepted paradigms in family medicine is that family physicians are principally involved in the management of people rather than pathologies.

There exists the tendency to explain family medicine in the terminology of traditional or biomedical medicine, to describe our method or process in terms of a scientific model that is inappropriate to most of our clinical activities. A more appropriate description is to say that, "symptom interpretation is very important; **only if** we take into account the personality, the defense mechanisms, the culture and the psychosocial circumstances of the patient – not to mention the doctor's personality and attitudes as well as the relationship that exists between doctor and patient. In other words, compared to the other specialist disciplines, we maintain that we have a unique way of **interpreting symptoms**. Therefore it is these "only ifs" that are the crux of our discipline's unique method and consequently our clinical competence.

In order to function within the framework of any discipline, its method or process must be adhered to. In medicine, this includes an accepted systematic procedure for gathering information and the rules needed for classifying, analyzing and validating that information. As family medicine is a scientific discipline, its method must adhere to principles of a scientific paradigm.

Our method is rooted in Engel's philosophy who melded three major scientific models of Newton, Einstein and The General Systems Theory into a holistic model and it advances the biopsychosocial paradigm as the valid basis for the practice of family medicine in West Africa.

This view is in consonance with Newtonian physics which maintains that a symptom is an objective reality, furthermore, that it has on objective identity and a meaning of its own. A further tenet of this model is that the observer of these symptoms (i.e. the doctor) is objective as well. Thus any number of doctors with equal knowledge and skills given the same set of symptom, regardless of the patients from whom they emanate, should come to exactly the same interpretation or diagnosis. Newtonian physics implies that what happens between the observed and the doctor-patient relationship is irrelevant.

Family Medicine has labeled the method associated with traditional Newtonian Medicine as "doctor-centered" or "disease-centered" and that of Family Medicine Einsteinian (patient-centered).

GEORGE ENGEL'S LEGACY

The late George Engel believed that to understand and respond adequately to patients' suffering – and to give them a sense of being understood – doctors must attend simultaneously to the **biological, psychological**, and **social** dimensions of illness as supported by the general systems theory. These are the 3 areas in which the biopsychosocial model was offered as a "new medical paradigm".

THREE CAUSES OF DE-HUMANIZING CARE IN MEDICINE

Three main strands in medical thinking have been identified as being responsible for dehumanizing care. Dualism, Reductionism and Detached observation.

DUALISM-THE SEPARATION OF BODY AND MIND

First, the dualistic nature of the biomedical model, with its separation of body and mind included an implicit privileging of the former (body) as more "real" and therefore more worthy of a scientific clinician's attention. Engel rejected this view for encouraging physicians to maintain a strict separation between the body-as-machine and the narrative biography and emotions of the person – to focus on the disease to the exclusion of the person who was suffering – without building bridges between the two realms.

Engel research in psychosomatics pointed toward a more integrative view, showing that fear, rage, neglect, and attachment had physiologic and developmental effects on the whole organism.

REDUCTIONISM

Second, Engel criticized the excessively materialistic and reductionist orientation of medical thinking. According to these principles, anything that could not be objectively verified and explained at the level of cellular and molecular processes was ignored or devalued.

Engel's perspective is contrasted with a so-called monistic or reductionist view, in which all phenomena could be reduced to smaller parts and understood as molecular interactions. For instance; fever ↔ plasmodium ↔ malaria.

The main focus of this criticism – a cold, impersonal, technical, biomedically-oriented style of clinical practice – may not have been so much a matter of underlying philosophy, but discomfort with practice that neglected the human dimension of suffering.

THE DETACHED OBSERVER

The third element was the influence of the observer on the observed. Engel understood that one cannot understand a system from the inside without disturbing the system in some way; in other words, in the human dimension, as in the world of particle physics, one cannot assume a stance of pure objectivity. In that way, Engel provided a rationale for including the human dimension of the physician and the patient as a legitimate focus for scientific study.

Rather, it may be that the content and emotions that constitute the doctor's relationship with the patient are the fundamental principles of biopsychosocial-oriented clinical practice, which then inform the manner in which the doctor exercises his or her power.

Nor did he endorse a holistic-energetic view, many of whose adherents spouse a biopsychosocial philosophy; these views hold that all physical phenomena are ephemeral and controllable by the manipulation of healing energies.

SYSTEMS THINKING IN THE BIOPYSCHOSOCIAL METHOD

In embracing Systems Theory, Engel recognized that mental and social phenomena depended upon but could not necessarily be, explained in terms of more basic physical phenomena given our of knowledge.

He endorsed what would now be considered a **complexity view**, in which different levels of the biopsychosocial hierarchy could interact, but the rules of interaction might not be directly derived from the rules of the higher and lower rungs of the biopsychosocial ladder. Instead, they would be considered emergent properties that would be highly dependent on the persons involved and the initial conditions with which they were presented.

THE BIOPSYCHOSOCIAL MODEL AND RELATIONSHIP-CENTERED CARE

The practical application of the biopsychosocial model, which is called **biopsychosocially oriented clinical practice,** does not necessarily evolve from the constructs of interactional dualism or circular causality.

FOCUS

The basic principles of the biopsychosocial model according to the emotional tone that engraves the relationship with such characteristics as caring, trustworthiness, and openness.

PILLARS OF THE BIOPSYCHOSOCIAL MODEL

- Self-awareness
- Self-calibration as a way to reduce bias
- Educating the emotions to assist with diagnosis and forming therapeutic relationships;
- An emotional style characterized by empathic curiosity
- Active cultivation of trust
- Using informed intuition
- Communicating clinical evidence to foster dialogue, not just the mechanical application of protocol.

SELF-AWARENESS: SELF AUDITING

The physician must be capable of an ongoing self-audit simply because his or her performance is never the same from moment to moment. It is a deliberative and sometimes frankly physician-centered approach so it is not without` its perils; however some authors regard this constant vigilance as a fundamental requirement for professions that require high reliability in the face of unexpected events.

In the practice of self-awareness and self-auditing, the physician must practice mindfulness in everyday practice by the habits of attentive observation, critical curiosity, informed flexibility, and presence which underlies the physician's ability to self-monitor, be vigilant, and respond with compassion.

CALIBRATING THE PHYSICIAN: SELF-CALIBRATION AS A WAY TO REDUCE BIAS

The biopsychosocial model calls for expanding the number and types of habits to be consciously learned and objectively monitored to maintain the centrality of the patient. The doctor is in some ways like a musical instrument that needs to be calibrated, tuned, and adjusted to perform adequately. For instance the **physician's skills** should be judged on their ability to produce greater health or to relieve the patient's suffering – whether they include creating an adequate emotional tone, gathering an accurate history, or distinguishing between what the patient needs and what the patient says he or she wants. In that regard, a clinical skill includes the **ethical mandate** not only to find out what concerns the patient, but to bring the physician's agenda to the table and influence the patient's behavior. Sometimes doing so may include uncovering psychosocial correlates of otherwise unexplained somatic symptoms (such as ongoing abuse or alcoholism) to break the cycle of medicalization and iatrogenesis.

To abandon this obligation, is breaking an implicit social contract between physicians and society.

Recognizing Bias: The grounding of medical decisions based on scientific evidence, while also integrating the clinician's professional experience, is now a well-accepted tenet of the founders of the evidence-based medicine movement. However, the method for the incorporation of experience has not been well described than the method for judging the quality of scientific evidence. For example, doctors should learn how their decisions might be biased by the ethnic group and sex of the patient, among other factors, and also the tendency to close the case prematurely to rid oneself of the burden of attempting to solve complex problems.

Educating the Emotions: to assist with diagnosis and forming therapeutic relationships.

There are methods for emotional education, just as there are for learning new knowledge and skills. By receiving a hostile patient with respect it clarifies for the clinician that the patient's emotions are the patient's – and not the physician's – and also sets the stage for the patient to reflect as well. Similarly, the physician must know how to recognize and when to express his or her own emotions, sometimes setting limits and boundaries in the interest of preserving a functional relationship.

Tolerance of uncertainty, for example, is amenable to observation and calibration – making decisions in the absence of complete information is a characteristic of an expert practitioner, in contrast to the technician who views his role as simply following protocols.

Cultivating Curiosity: An emotional style characterized by empathic curiosity

The next step in the application of clinical evidence to medical care is the cultivation of curiosity.

Thus, cultivated naivete is considered one of the fundamental habits characteristic of experienced doctor. Another aspect of this emotional tone is an empathic curiosity about the patient as person. This empathic curiosity allows the doctor to maintain an open mind and not to consider that any case is ever closed. If the patient does not surprise us today, perhaps he or she will tomorrow. It is the capacity for expecting the unexpected, just as if the physician were another doctor seeing the patient for the first time.

There is also an ethical component of this emotional tone – there are no "good" or "bad" patients, nor are there "interesting" and "boring" diseases. Patients should not have to legitimize their suffering by describing only illnesses that make the clinician feel comfortable or confident.

Creating Trust: Active cultivation of trust

The expert clinician considers explicitly, as a core skill, the achievement in the encounter of an emotional tone conducive to a therapeutic relationship.

For that reason, all consultations might be judged on the basis of cordiality, optimism, genuineness, and good humor.

Using Informed Intuition

The role of intuition is central. Just as some authors maintain that professional competence is based in tacit, rather than explicit, knowledge, expertise often is manifest in insights that are difficult to track on a strictly cognitive level.

If a clinician, encountering a situation in which he normally would use a particular treatment, has the intuition, for a reason that has not yet become clear, that treatment might not be the best for this particular patient, it can be suggested, rather than considering it a feeling from nowhere that might be discarded, perhaps the intuition can later be traced to a set of concrete observations about the patient that were not easy for the clinician to describe at the time.

That these observations often are manifest only when cases are reviewed after the fact does not diminish the ethical obligation that the clinician use all of his or her capabilities, including those which cannot be readily explained.

Communicating Clinical Evidence

Evidence should be communicated in terms the patient can understand, in small digestible pieces, at a rate at which it can be assimilated. Information overload may have two effects – reduction incomprehension and increasing the emotional distance between physician and patient. Communication of clinical evidence should foster understanding, not simply answers.

Further Development of the Biopsychosocial Model

George Engel formulated the biopsychosocial model as a dynamic, interactional, but dualistic (not to be confused with dualism i.e. separation of mind and body) view of human experience in which there is mutual influence of mind and body. Added to that model the need to balance a circular model of causality with the need to make linear approximations (especially in planning treatments) and the need to change the clinician's stance from objective detachment to reflective participation, thus infusing care with greater warmth and caring.

The biopsychosocial model was not so much a paradigm shift – in the sense of a crisis of the scientific method in medicine or the elaboration of new scientific laws – as it was an expanded application of existing knowledge to the needs of each patient.

In the 35 years that have elapsed since Engel first proposed the biopsychosocial model, two new intellectual trends have emerged that could make it even more robust.

First, we can move beyond the problematic issue of mind-body duality by recognizing that knowledge is socially constructed. To some extent, such categories as "mind" or "body" are of our own creation. They are useful to the extent that they focus our thinking and action in helpful ways (e.g. they contribute to health, well-being, and efficient use of resources), but when taken too literally, they can also entrap and limit us by creating boundaries that need not exist. Therefore, by maintaining "fragile" or "fluid" categories, we can alter or dispose of these categories as new evidence accumulates or when there is a need to engage in flexible, out-of-the-box thinking.

Second, we can move beyond the multidimensional and multifactorial **linear** thinking to consider complexity theory as a more adequate model for understanding causality, dualism, and participation in care. Complexity theory shows how, in open systems, it is often impossible to know all of the contributors to and influences on particular health outcomes. By describing the ways in which systems tend to self-organize, it provides guideposts to inform the clinician's actions. It also buffers the tendency to impose unrealistic expectations that one can know and control all of these contributors and influences.

George Engel's most enduring contribution was to broaden the scope of the clinician's gaze.

The BIOPSYCHOSOCAL model in practice - Exploring both the disease and the illness experience

The disease is a diagnostic label given by the physician; the illness is the practical experience of symptoms, feelings, weaknesses, discomforts, attitudes, and impairment of relationships by the patient. It represents personal, interpersonal, and cultural reactions to discomfort and sickness. The family physician must investigate illness as well as disease, and direct clinical care at both. The biopsychosocial model is both a philosophy of clinical care and a practical clinical guide.

Philosophically, it is a way of understanding how suffering, disease, and illness are affected by multiple levels of organization, from the social to the molecular. At the practical level, it is a way of understanding the patient's subjective experience as an essential contributor to accurate diagnosis, health outcomes, and human care.

Engel's biopsychosocial model was a call to change our way of understanding the patient and to expand the domain of medical knowledge to address the needs of each patient. It is perhaps the transformation of the way illness, suffering, and healing as well as the various causes and factors that influence them are viewed by physicians that may be Engel's most durable contribution to Family Medicine.

Structural Causality: In contrast to the circular view, structural causality describes a hierarchy of unidirectional cause-effect relationships – necessary causes, precipitants, sustaining forces, and associated events.

For instance, a necessary cause for tuberculosis is a mycobacterium, precipitants can be a low body temperature, and a sustaining force a low caloric intake. Complexity science can facilitate understanding of a clinical situation, but most of the time a structural model is what guides practical action. For example, if we think that Mr. J is hypertensive because he consumes too much salt, has a stressful job, poor social supports, and an over-responsible personality type, following a circular causal model, possibly all of these factors are truly contributory to his high blood pressure. But, when we suggest to him that he take an antihypertensive medication, or that he consume less salt, or that he take a stress-reduction course, or that he see a psychotherapist to reduce his sense of guilt, we are creating an implicit hierarchy of causes.

Causal attributions have the power to create reality and transform the patient's view of his/her own world. The attribution of causality can be used to blame the patient for his or her illness ("If only he had not smoked so much...."), and also may have the power of suggestion and might actually worsen the patient's condition ("Everytime there is a fight, your dizziness worsens, don't you see?").

A doctor who listens well might agree when a patient worries that a family argument precipitated a myocardial infarction; although this interpretation may have meaning to the patient, it is inadequate as a total explanation of why the patient suffered a myocardialinfarction.

There is therefore the need for a subsequent **hierarchy of decisions** of which cause has the greatest likely contribution to his high blood pressure must be created. Which would be most responsive to our actions? What is the added value of this action, after having done others? Which strategy will give the greatest result with the least harm and with the least expenditure of resources?

The Comprehensive Biopsychosocial Assessment

The comprehensive assessment, (sometimes called the 3-stage assessment), is an extremely useful tool for a holistic approach to patient problems and their management.

The comprehensive assessment is a statement of each of the patient's problems taken as far as the available information allows. It is considered in 3 stages based on the Biopsychosocial aspects of patient care:

Clinical assessment: A statement of the disease entity, as far as the available information allows.

Individual assessment: This includes everything about the patient which has bearing on the clinical assessment.

Contextual Assessment: This includes everything external to the patient which has bearing on the clinical assessment.

The Complete Biopsychosocial Assessment Profile

ASSESSMENT	SUB-SECTION	DETAILS
CLINICAL (Bio..)	Anatomical	• Which Structure / organ is affected
	Pathological	• What Pathological process
	Aetiological	• Cause
	Functional	• What disability or dysfunction does the condition cause?
INDIVIDUAL (..psycho..)	Personal factors	• Age, sex, occupation etc.
	Patient's thoughts	• Understanding of the condition
	Patient's feelings	• Fears, guilt etc.
	Patient's expectations	• From the consultation; of the doctor; of himself
	Behavioural diagnosis (Why patient came)	• Limit of tolerance • Limit of anxiety • Problems of living • Signal behaviour • Opportunity • Administrative reasons • No disease
CONTEXTUAL (..social..)	Immediate	• At home • Family & friends
	Work & activities	• At work, or school • Sport & clubs
	Community	• Neighbourhood • Religion • Cultural factors
	Social classification	• Loss • Stress

CHAPTER 6

SOCIAL SUPPORT AND FAMILY FUNCTIONING

Ewedairo O. A., Attoye T. E.

S OCIAL SUPPORT IS one of the most well-documented psychosocial factors influencing physical health outcomes. Social support is the perception and actuality that one is cared for, has assistance available from other people, and that one is part of a supportive social network. Support can come from many sources, including but not limited to family, friends, romantic partners, organization, co-workers.

FORMS OF SOCIAL SUPPORT:

Mattson et al. describes five forms of social support which are generally used by researchers they include:

Emotional support: this is the offering of empathy, concern, affection, love, trust, acceptance, intimacy, encouragement, or caring. It is the warmth and nurturance provide by sources of social support. Providing emotional support can let the individual know that he or she is valued.

Esteem Support: this is the form of support that bolsters an individual's self-esteem or beliefs in their ability to handle problems or perform needed tasks.

Tangible support: this is the provision of financial assistance, material goods, or services. Also called instrumental support, this form of social support encompasses the concrete, direct ways people assist others.

Informational support: this is the provision of advice, guidance, suggestion, or useful information to someone. This type of information has the potential to help others solve problems.

Network support: this is the type of support that gives some a sense of social belonging and reminds them of availability of support from the network. Social support can be measured in terms of structural support or functional support. Structural support (also called social integration) refers to the extent to which a recipient is connected within a social network, like the number of social ties or how integrated a person is within his or her social network. Family relationships, friends, and membership in clubs and organizations contribute to social integration. Functional support looks at the specific functions that members in this social network can provide, such as the emotional, instrumental and informational support.

For the purpose of research, social support is also commonly divided into perceived and received support. Perceived support refers to a recipient's subjective judgment that providers will offer (or have offered) effective help during times of need. Received support (also called enacted support) refers to specific supportive actions (e.g., advice or reassurance) offered by providers during times of need which matches the types of support sought by the recipient. Perceived support has been more consistently related to beneficial health outcomes than has received support.

SOCIAL SUPPORT AND HEALTH:

There are two general theoretical models that propose processes through which social relationships/social support may influence health: the stress buffering and main effects models.

The buffering hypothesis suggests that social relationships may provide resources (informational, emotional, or tangible) that promote adaptive behavioural or neuroendocrine responses to acute or chronic stressors (e.g., illness, life events, life transitions). From this perspective, the term social support is used to refer to the real or perceived availability of social resources.

The main effects model proposes that social relationships may associated with protective health effects through more direct means, such as cognitive, emotional, behavioural, and biological influences that are not explicitly intended as help or support. For instance, social relationships may directly encourage or indirectly model healthy behaviours; thus, being part of a social network is typically associated with conformity to social norms relevant to health and self-care. In addition, being part of a social network gives individuals meaningful roles that provide self-esteem and purpose to life.

Biological Pathways of Social Support and Health:

Attempts have been made to identify bio-psychosocial pathways for the link between social support and health. Social support has been found to positively impact the immune, neuroendocrine, and cardiovascular systems.

Immune system: social support is generally associated with better immune function. Of particular note, social support is associated with higher levels of natural killer cell activity and natural killer cells are thought to play an important "surveillance" role in cancer. Also being more socially integrated is correlated with lower levels of inflammation (as measured by Creative protein, a marker of inflammation), and people with more social support have a lower susceptibility to the common cold.

Neuroendocrine system: social support has been linked to lower cortisol ("stress hormone") levels in response to stress. Cortisol like other steroids is known to be and immunosuppressant. Also a perception of partner support was uniformly associated with higher oxytocin levels which are associated with decrease cortisol level. Neuroimaging work has found that social support decreases activation of regions in the brain associated with social distress, and that this diminished activity was also related to lowered cortisol levels.

Cardiovascular system: social support has been found to lower cardiovascular reactivity to stressors. Social support may thus be beneficial because it "buffers" the potentially harmful influences of stress-induced cardiovascular reactivity. Social support has also been found to lower blood pressure and heart rates during everyday life, which are known to benefit the cardiovascular system. Thus individuals with low levels of social support have higher mortality rates, especially from cardiovascular disease.

Others: there are several other areas of health where social support have been shown to be beneficial, for instance social support is considered a key component of behavioural weight-loss programs, it has been shown to help in weight loss interventions and weight loss maintenance, Kiernan et al. reported that women who "never" experienced family support were least likely to lose weight (45.7% lost weight) whereas women who experienced both frequent friend and support were more likely to lose weight (71.6% lost weight). This study relied on self-report to determine support received, this may however be affected by emotions at the time of data collection, however being a randomized trial would have reduced the risk of differential misclassification which could have occurred.

Smoking cessation was also mediated by social support from group therapy which was found to be superior to individual therapy. A Cochrane review reports that group therapy offers individuals the opportunity to learn behavioural techniques for smoking cessation, and to provide each other with mutual support.

Social support has also been shown to help improve adherence to medications. DiMatteo, shown in a meta-analysis of 122 studies with remarkable consistency a positive correlation between social support and adherence to medication. He suggested that assistance and support from friends and family have been implicated in promoting patient adherence by encouraging optimism, self-esteem and buffering the stresses of being ill. Social support also decreases the length of hospitalization after heart surgery.

Social support and birth outcomes: studies have suggested that lack of, or poor social support during pregnancy may lead to the birth of small for gestational age/LBW babies. Dejin-Karlsson et al in Sweden in their prospective cohort study, found that women with a low degree of participation in society and those lacking instrumental support (access to advice and information) shared the greatest risk of giving birth to small for gestational age babies, they concluded that lack of psychosocial resources, such as social stability, social participation, emotional and instrumental support, all increased the likelihood of delivering an infant that was small for gestational age.

Morhason-Bello et al. in Ibadan reported that social support also decreased the rate of caesarean section and the duration of labour. A randomized control trial in Nigeria also showed that social support helped reduced the time from birth to initiation of breast feeding amongst first time mothers. The study revealed that women who had a companion of their choice in the delivery room had all initiated breast feeding within 26minutes of giving birth while none of the control group had done likewise after 30minutes of giving birth with some not initiating breast feeding even after 12 hours of giving birth.

A Cochrane review of randomized controlled trials reported that women who had continuous support during child birth were more likely to have a spontaneous vaginal birth and less likely to have intra-partum analgesia. In addition their labours were shorter, they were less likely to have a caesarean section or instrumental vaginal birth, regional analgesia or a baby with a low 5-minute Apgar score. Social support in general has also been shown to help patients to adapt better to diseases.

Though many benefits have been found, not all research indicates positive effects of social support on these systems. Some people may experience "negative" social support which may influence unhealthy habits of cigarette smoking, decreased physical activity and alcohol consumption all of which may have negative effect on the health.

It has been suggested that women benefit more from social support than men possibly because women tend to have more emotionally intimate relationships. It can thus be inferred from this that women may therefore feel the negative effect of absent or negative social support more than men.

MEASURES OF SOCIAL SUPPORT:

Several tools for the measurement of social support have been developed, each of the tools have different psychometric properties, strengths and weaknesses. Some of the measures of social support include, Arizonal Social Support Interview, Duke-UNC Functional Social Support Questionnaire – DUFSS, Medical Outcome Study: Social Support Survey – MOS- SSS, Multidimensional Scale of Perceived Social Support – MSPSS, Norbeck Social Support Questionnaire – NSSQ, Perceived Social Support Scale, - PSSS, Social Support Questionnaire – SSQ etc.

According to an extensive review by Lopez et al., the 4 social support measures that had the strongest documented psychometric support are; Medical Outcomes Study: Social Support Survey – MOS-SSS, The Social Provisions Scale – SPS, Duke-UNC Functional Social Support Questionnaire – DUFSS and Multidimensional Scale of perceived Social Support – MSPSS.

MOS-SSS

The Medical Outcomes Study: Social Support Survey (MOS-SSS) is relatively brief (either the original 19 item version or the 12 item abbreviated version) measure of social support. It assesses four components of perceived availability of social support, including (1) emotional support/informational support, (2) tangible support (including material support), (3) positive social interaction (does person have friends that are available to have fun), and (4) affectionate support (including loving and nurturing relationships).

Strengths of MOS-SSS:

Measure assesses multiple facets of social support and the subscales maybe used separately.

Measure is free and easily accessible, it has solid psychometrics for many of the samples on which the measure has been used and has been used with culturally and linguistically diverse populations, both in the U.S. and other countries, including mothers of very young children.

Weaknesses of MOS-SSS:

The measure does not evaluate the level of strain experienced within the social support network. The strain may affect how, to what extent, or when social support is available to the respondent. Measure was not designed specifically to tap parents' experiences with, or needs for, social support and measure does not capture information on specific sources of, or satisfaction with social support.

SPS:

The SPS assesses six dimensions of social support received within the context of interpersonal relationships: (1) Guidance (receiving advice and/or information), (2) Reliable alliance (feeling assured that one can rely on certain others for concrete assistance if necessary), (3) Reassurance of worth (feeling important to or valued by others), (4) Opportunity for nurturance (feeling needed to provide nurturing attention to others), (5) attachments (receiving a sense of emotional security from close relationships), and (6) Social integration (feeling a sense of belonging in a group, which includes others with similar interests, values, or ideas).

Strengths of the SPS:

Measure is easily accessible from the authors and scoring in simple and straight forward. Scores from individual subscales or global support score may be used. Measure has had some use with non-Caucasian samples, both in the U.S. and in Spain. Measure captures taps multiple dimensions of personal relationships, in a brief survey and solid psychometrics exist for many of the samples on which the measure has been used.

Weaknesses of the SPS:

This measure does not collect information about the size of the respondent's social support network. Without this information, it is unclear how tenuous or reliable the network might be if even one important relationship is lost or damaged. The measure does not evaluate the level of strain experienced within the social support network. The strain may affect how, to what extent, or when social support is available to the respondent and the measure does not directly assess tangible or concrete support.

DUFSS:

The Duke-UNC Functional Social Support Questionnaire (DUFSS) is the shortest (8items) of the 4 recommended measures of social support. The scale assesses the amount and type of perceived emotional social support, including: (1) Confidant Support (having someone to talk to, social with, receive advice from) (2) Affective Support (being shown live and affection). A 10-item adapted version developed by the Consortium for Longitudinal Studies of Child Abuse and Neglect studies, or LONGSCAN added 3 additional items related to instrumental support, including assistance with transportation, assistance with cooking or household tasks, and help caring for a child. The overall psychometric properties of the original DUFSS were somewhat modest, but somewhat stronger when including the studies conducted with the 10item adapted LONGSCAN version.

Strengths of the DUFSS:

The measure is very brief, the original and adapted versions of the measure have been used with parents and adaptations of the scale have demonstrated evidence for establishing concurrent validity.

Weaknesses of DUFSS:

The evidence for establishing the measure's concurrent validity is not very strong. The correlations between the DUFSS and the social activities measures are low, though statistically significant and most of the studied that have used the DUFSS have modified it, which lends difficulty to interpreting and comparing psychometrics across studies and the measure neither captures the specific sources of social support nor provides information about the size of the social support network.

Multidimensional Scale of Perceived Social Support [MSPSS]

MSPSS was developed by Zimet et al. in 1988. The MSPSS measures perceived adequacy of social support from 3 sources: family (items 3, 4, 8, and 1), friends (items 6, 7, 9, and 12), and significant other (items 1, 2, 5, and 10). Twelve-item ratings are made on a 7-point Likert-type scale ranging from very strongly disagree (1) to very strongly agree (7). The total score possible range between 12 and 84. The participants are classified as having high, moderate or low perceived social support if they had scores of between 69-84, and 12-48 respectively. MSPSS rather than capturing differences in the types of perceived social support as the MOS-SSS does, the MSPSS captures variability in the 3 major sources of support.

Strengths of MSPSS:

Brief, 12 items tool, results indicated that comprehension of MSPSS items requires only a fourth-grade reading level. It captures multiple aspects of perceived social support, across 3 major sources of support (Family, Friends or Significant Others). It uses the term "special person," rather than "significant other" within the Significant Other subscale; this allows participants to respond to the items, whether or not the participants have a romantic partner and there is established evidence for reliability, for total score and the 3 subscales.

This measure of social support has been validated for use in South Africa and has also been adapted and validated in Uganda.

Weakness of MSPSS:

Hasn't has a lot of work done with families and/or parents of young children. The MSPSS was used for this research because of the simplicity of the tool, it measures social support across different dimensions, the language is simple and easy to understand and the tool has been validated in 2 African countries and found to have sound psychometric properties.

FAMILY AND FAMILY FUNCTION:

Physicians can no longer think of health as simply an individual issue. Humans are social beings, and their health is strongly influenced by the social context, especially social relationships. The family is the most intimate current and past social environment, the family has a powerful influence on health beliefs and behaviours and on overall mental and physical health. Illness in the family affects family relationships and the health of other family members.

The family, according to the United State Census Bureau, is defined as a householder and one or more other people living in the same household who are related to the householder by birth, marriage, or adoption.

FAMILY INFLUENCE ON HEALTH

Genetic: the family influences health in several ways and are a major source of support to a patient. The important way the family affects health is through genetics, several diseases are transmitted through families. For instance, asthma a chronic respiratory disease can run in families. Diabetes, hypertension and breast cancer are other diseases with genetic predisposition.

Health promotion: the family can also be a resource for health promotion. Unhealthy behaviours account for much of morbidity or suffering from chronic illnesses, such as heart disease, cancer diabetes, and stroke. Health habits usually develop, are maintained, and are changed within the context of the family. Unhealthy behaviours or risk factors tend to cluster within families, because family members tend to share similar diets, physical activities, and use or abuse of unhealthy substances such as smoking.

For instance the family has been shown to be able to influence persons trying to quit smiling either positively or negatively. Koshy et al. in Scotland reported in a research on pregnant women in a smoking cessation programme, that women who quit smoking during pregnancy talked more about receiving active praise/encouragement than those who did not from partners, family and friends. This was a qualitative case control study of quitters and non-quitters, however, the sample size of 12 in each group was small therefore reducing the power of the study. Hill et al. in Washington in another relatively large prospective study reported that parent smoking contributes to the onset of daily smoking in their teenagers even if parents practice good family management, hold norms against teen tobacco use, and do not involve their children in their own tobacco use. Because of these types of research findings, it is being suggested that the family be included in smoking cessation programmes. In the area of dental hygiene as well, the family plays a key role, it has been reported that parents' dental health habits influence their children's oral health. Families are therefore key components of health promotion strategies.

Access to healthcare: the family also determines access to health care services in various ways; family structure, the level of education in the family socio-economic status of the family, cultural beliefs and practices all influence the health seeking behaviours and access to health care within the family.

Spread of diseases: The family plays an important role in the spreading of diseases and conversely can help prevent the spread of diseases. HIV, malaria, conjunctivitis, tuberculosis etc. are communicable diseases that can rapidly spread within the family. As highlighted above, non-communicable diseased such as cardiovascular diseases, breast cancer, diabetes etc. can also spread within families as well. Recognizing the role the family plays in the propagation of disease states is key to planning preventive strategies and they (the family) must be incorporated into preventive programmes.

The family as care givers: The families act as the care givers and are the source of support especially when it comes to chronic illnesses in a family member. Bray et al., affirm that the "families, not health care providers, are the primary caretakers for patients with chronic illness". They are the ones who help with most of the physical demands of the illness, ranging from preparing special meals for a family member with heart disease to assisting with insulin injections for a diabetic to changing adult diapers and emptying colostomy bags. How well the family copes and adapts to a chronic illness has a major influence on the course of the illness (i.e., pathogenic model) to examining ways in which families influence, positively or negatively, the course of chronic illness.

Family caregivers are essential members of the health care team. They provide clinical observation, direct care, case management, and a range of other services, to achieve the positive effects of the family on health, the family must be "functional".

FAMILY FUNCTIONING

The need to enhance family functioning to improve the health status of children and parents os increasingly recognized. Family functioning has become an important public health issue because it is associated with a range of child health and wellbeing indicators, including physical and mental health, risk behaviours, and developmental, academic, and social outcomes.

Family functioning generally refers to interactions with family members that involve physical, emotional, and psychological activities and affects many aspects of family life including acceptance of individuals, consensus on decisions, communication, and the ability to solve day-to-day problems.

Family functioning can also be described as a family system process used to provide the biological, psychological, social development and maintenance of family members. It typically includes such areas as communication, beliefs, cohesion, adaptability, structure, relation quality, parenting style, task accomplishment, competence, conflict, and problem solving.

Healthy Family Functioning:

According to the World Health Organization, "healthy family functioning" is defined in terms of a family unit (however it is conceived in any given culture) effectively coping with cultural, environmental, psychosocial, and socioeconomic stresses throughout the family life cycle Healthy/Positive family functioning is characterized by emotional closeness, warmth, support and security, well-communicated and consistently applied age-appropriate expectations, stimulating and educational interactions, the cultivation and modeling of physical health promotion strategies, high quality relationships between all family members and involvement of family members in community activities.

There are many different opinions as to which form of family functions is the best, however, regardless of structure, there is a well-established consensus that families which function well have most of the following characteristics:

- ❖ Parents who model healthy lives to their children.
- ❖ Family members have some independence from each other (e.g. a young person is not obliged to feel, think or behave in a prescribed manner on all issues or in all circumstances)
- ❖ Parents actively build self-esteem in their children through compliments and demonstrating affection.
- ❖ Family members actively listen to each other.
- ❖ Family members argue without wounding each other (i.e. no personal attacks, but stick to the merits of an argument).
- ❖ The family participates in activities that all members enjoy.
- ❖ The family places value on reciprocal support.
- ❖ Parents spend time with their children.
- ❖ Parents are reliable and trustworthy, but not so predictable that they are taken for granted.

Unhealthy Family Functioning:

Unhealthy/dysfunctional family functioning is said to exist in a family when conflict, misbehaviour, reduced parental monitoring and management of children's behavior and often child neglect or abuse on the part of individual parents occur continually and regularly, leading other members to accommodate such actions.

Dysfunctional families have one or more of the following family pathologies,

- ❖ Keeping the family "secrets."
- ❖ Being unable to identify and express feelings.
- ❖ Playing one family member against the other (intrafamily hostility).
- ❖ Perfectionism.
- ❖ The inability to play, have fun, and be spontaneous (rigidity).
- ❖ Double messages.
- ❖ A high tolerance for inappropriate behavior.
- ❖ Having identities of individuals overlapping with others.

The beneficial effects of family on health as listed above are seen when there is healthy family functioning, conversely, when there is unhealthy family functioning, several adverse effects are also observed.

For instance, dysfunctional family systems can promote and maintain alcoholism. In a study by Schafer in New Zealand, he found that all participants in his study population felt they had been unable to develop functional relationships with either their family-of-origin or current family members and they identified a strong connection between these dysfunctional family relationships and their subsequent substance abuse. He also reported that first-degree relatives of alcoholics are three to five times more likely to develop alcoholism than the general population. The study was a qualitative study with 12 participants who had about one hour semi-structured interviews and findings were transcribed. This methodology has some challenges as respondents tend to provide responses they believe the interviewer sought.

Unhealthy family functioning was also found to be associated with the development of emotional and behavioural problems.

Abu-Rayya et al. reported that unhealthy family functioning increased significantly the risks for emotional problems, peer problems, conduct problems, and substantially increased the risk for overall emotional and behavioural problems among Australian children aged 4-15 years.

Shek in a study done on Chinese adolescents, found that family functioning was significantly related to measures of adolescent psychological well-being (existential well-being, life satisfaction, self-esteem, sense of mastery, general psychiatric morbidity), school adjustment (perceived academic performance, satisfaction with academic performance, and school conduct), and problem behavior (delinquent and substance abuse behavior).

Also the development of obesity has also been linked to family functioning. Dinsmore et al. in Oregon USA, found that eating habits, behaviours and attitudes which in turn determines the presence or absence of obesity was associated with family functioning. While another study showed that poorer family functioning scores are correlated with greater body mass index (BMI) in fifth-grade children.

DETERMINING FAMILY FUNCTION:

The importance of family and family function on physical and psychological health of individuals is apparent, it is therefore important in family practice that the family function of patients seen in this setting be assessed when possible especially when the family will be involved in the care of the patient. Several approaches to examining and characterizing family function for research purposes have proposed, these include a combination of analysis of communication, observation of interaction, and individual patient report. Many of these approaches are however time-consuming and not practical for use in large sample studies requiring a brief instrument and are nit feasible for use in the family practice setting.

For instance the Family Assessment Measure (FAM) assesses family function across three levels; whole family system (general scale with fifty items), various dyadic relationship (dyadic scale with forth two items) and individual functioning (self-rating scale forty two items). This is a 134item tool which cannot feasible be used for large scale research or a busy family practice setting.

Some tools used for assessing family functioning in a clinic setting include; family Adaptability and Cohesion Evaluation Scale (FACES), Family APGAR and the McMaster Family Assessment Device (FAD) with FAD being the most common tool being used.

McMaster Family Assessment Device:

The Family Assessment Device (FAD) is a self-administered measure based on the McMaster Model of Family Functioning (MMFF) and "describes the structural and organizational properties of the family group and the patterns of transactions among family members". It was developed by Epstein, et al. in 1983.

The measure consists of seven scales including a General Functioning scale which incorporates items from each of the other scales to assess the overall level of family functioning. The remaining six scales assess the six dimensions of the MMFF which include:

1. **Problem Solving:** this assesses the family's ability to solve problems at a level that maintains family functioning.
2. **Communication:** this assesses whether the verbal messages that are exchanges between family members are "clear with respect to the content and direct in the sense that the person spoken to is the person to whom the message is intended".
3. **Roles:** this assesses whether the family has organized patterns of behavior for operating family functions which include: "provision of resources, providing nurturance and support, supporting personal development, maintaining and managing the family systems and providing adult sexual gratification". Also, assessment of Roles includes consideration of assigned

tasks within the family and whether they are carried out responsibly.

4. **Affective Responsiveness:** this assesses the degree to which family members express appropriate affect in the presence of a range of stimuli.

5. **Affective Involvement:** this assesses the degree to which family members are interested in and take value in other members' concerns.

6. **Behavior Control:** this assesses the way in which family member maintain standards of behavior within the family system.

The questionnaire is self-administered and each family member above the age of 12 years rates his or her agreement or disagreement of how the statement describes their family. Each of the 6 sub-scales has a set of items (53 in all) with 4 possible responses for each of the items each with a score; Strongly Agree=4, Agree=3, Disagree=2 and Strongly Disagree=1.

Using a guide provided by the developers, the total score of each of the sub-scales are determined and divided b7 the number of items on each sub-scale. Individual scales score range 1.0 (best functioning) to 4.0 (worst functioning).

FAD has been extensively used in research and found to be valid, and has been translated in 14 languages including French, Italian and Spanish. The 12 item general functioning scale of FAD can also be used alone for rapid assessment of overall family functioning.

Family Adaptability and Cohesion Evaluation Scale (FACES):

The Family Adaptability and Cohesion Scale (FACES) was developed in 1979 by Olson et al. based on a "circumplex model" the circumplex model is based on 3 key concepts for understanding family functioning; Family cohesion, flexibility (adaptability) and communication.

Family Cohesion:

Cohesion is defined as the emotional bonding that exists between family members. There are four levels of cohesion ranging from disengaged (very low) to separated (low to moderate) to connected (moderate to high) to enmeshed (very high) (see figure 1). It is hypothesized that the central or balanced levels of cohesion (separated and connected) make for optimal family functioning.

Family adaptability/flexibility:

Adaptability is the family's ability to change its power structure, role relationships and rules to respond to situational or developmental needs. The four levels of flexibility range from rigid (very low) to structured (low to moderate) to flexible (moderate to high) to chaotic (very high) (see Figure 1). As with cohesion, it is hypothesized that central or balanced levels of flexibility (structured and flexible) are more conducive to good marital and family functioning, with the extremes (rigid and chaotic) being the most problematic for families as they move in the their life cycle.

Family Communication:

This is defined as the positive communication skills utilized in the couple or family system. Communication is the third dimension in the Circumplex Model and is considered a facilitating dimension. Communication is considered critical for facilitating movement on the other two dimensions. Because it is a facilitating dimension, communication is not graphically included in the model along with cohesion and flexibility. The most basic hypothesis derived from the Circumplex Model is that: couples and families with balanced types will generally function more adequately than those at the unbalanced types. Another hypothesis is that: balanced families will have more positive communication skills than unbalanced families.

The FACES tool is a self-administered questionnaire that assesses the responses of the family member along the flexibility and cohesion dimensions. Each statement offers a 5-point response which ranges from 'almost never', scoring 1, to 'almost always', scoring 5. The total score for questions on the cohesion and the adaptability dimensions are added and plotted on a grid and the overall family functioning whether balanced or unbalanced is determined.

There are currently four versions of the FACES tool available for research and they have varying degrees of complexities and validity. FACES IV was validated with 3 other tool, the family Assessment Device, Self-report Family Inventory and Family Satisfaction Scale.

Different versions of the FACES tool have been found to be useful for clinical research by different researchers; place et al. successfully used FACES II to categorize families of children who were fearful of attending schools and children with depressed parent(s) into flexibly enmeshed and rigidly disengaged families respectively while Joh et al. using FACES III found that adolescents with high adaptability and high cohesion showed low problem behaviours, Lehan et al. using the FACES IV reported that families of survivors of a traumatic brain injury had balanced adaptability and cohesion and they reported relatively high level of family communication and satisfaction.

Interestingly neither the FACES nor the McMaster FAD family assessment tool was found by the author to be used for research in West Africa or Nigeria.

FAMILY APGAR:

The Family APGAR assessment tool was developed by Smilkstein Gabriel in 1978 to elicit the patient's view of the functional state of his/her family. The tool comprises 5 questions which assess the patient's satisfaction with current family function and support provided by his/

her family. The five items are related to the following components of satisfaction with family function: adaptability, Partnership, Growth, Affection, and Resolve. The items were developed on the premise that a family member's perception of family functioning could be assessed by reported satisfaction with the five dimensions of family functioning listed above.

Definition of Family APGAR Components:

Adaptability: this is the utilization of intra and extra-familial resources for problem solving when the family equilibrium is stressed during a crisis.

Partnership: this is the sharing of decision making and nurturing responsibilities by the family members.

Growth: is the physical and emotional maturation and self-fulfillment that is achieved by the family members through mutual support and guidance.

Affection: is the caring or loving relationships that exist amongst family members.

Resolve: is the commitment to devote time to other members of the family for physical and emotional nurturing. It also usually involves the decision to share wealth and space.

Family APGAR and Clinical Practice:

Family APGAR's introduction into clinical practice was designed to provide a quick assessment of family functioning for the practicing physician. It was designed as an interviewer administered tool which can rapidly (less than 5 minutes) be used to assess the family functioning of an individual. A response format of three choices is provided: 2 = almost always, 1 = some of the time and 0 = hardly ever. Scores can range from 0 to 10, the higher the score the greater the respondent's satisfaction with his family functioning.

Mengel M, in 1987 decided to categorize the family APGAAR score, he recommended that anyone with a total score of 6 and below be categorized as having a dysfunctional family.

The score was further classified into moderately dysfunctional (poorly functional) and severely dysfunctional for scores 4-6 and 0-3 respectively, while a score of 7 and above represents a functional family.

It is recommended that Family APGAR scores from each member of a household be collected and the average score would represent the true family function of the family, it has however been suggested that an estimate of family satisfaction by the female head of the household will provide an accurate assessment of family functioning.

CHAPTER 7

THE UNCERTAINTY OF ILLNESS

I N STUDYING UNCERTAINTY in illness we draw parallels to certain concepts in physics. One is the Heisenberg Uncertainty Principle which states that you can never simultaneously know the exact position and the exact speed of an object because things in the universe behave like both a particle and a wave at the same time. The second is the observer effect which explains that the very act of observation causes changes in the phenomenon being observed.

Uncertainty in the context of medicine is the inability to determine the meaning of illness-related events, occurring when the decision maker is unable to assign definite value to objects or events, or is unable to predict outcomes accurately (Mishel, 1988). This encompasses questions about inconsistent test results, diagnoses, which treatments to pursue and even what foods to eat can consume a patient with worry (Spivey, 1997, p3).

Uncertainty is a constant occurrence from the diagnosis to living with a chronic illness. It decreases over time and returns on illness recurrence or exacerbation. Uncertainty is the most distressing to a person during the diagnosis phase. This is the place where health care providers could lessen the uncertainty on a patient by educating the patient about the illness, showing confidence in treated their illness, and giving the patient clear and concise information.

Studies regarding uncertainty date back to as early as 1960 by F. Davis. The beginning work gave some ideas about the relationship between ambiguity and a patient's psychological state. Mishel's work was the first to focus on uncertainty in illness. Mishel supported her models with research from not just the field of nursing but other related fields such as psychology. Health care providers can reduce uncertainty by providing information and being confident in their knowledge of the illness. Support from the patient's home or other patients helped to reduce a patient's anxiety level. A person's personality can also impact how they deal with being diagnosed with an illness. A more positive person may choose to look at their illness as an opportunity to reevaluate their life. A person whose view of life is more negative may experience a lower quality of life after their diagnosis. A more negative person may experience depression, anxiety, or a form of PTSD.

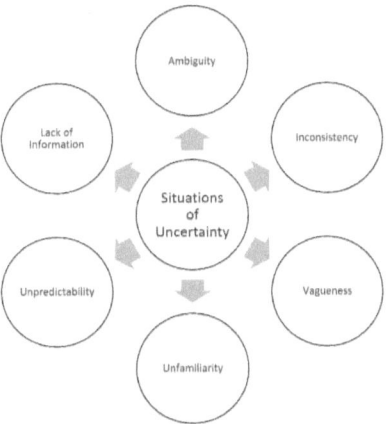

"A state of uncertainty is a major component of all illness experiences and it affects psychosocial adaptation and outcomes of disease".

Because the illness trajectory for the patient is complex, it is helpful to identify some situations that can cause uncertainty for the patient. These characteristics all have a direct relationship to the onset of uncertainty.

The theory of uncertainty of illness is composed of three major themes:

1. Antecedents of uncertainty- anything that occurs prior to the illness experience that affects the patient's thinking such as pain, prior experiences, and perception.
2. Appraisal of uncertainty- the process of placing a value on the uncertain situation.
3. Coping with uncertainty- activities that are used in dealing with the uncertainty.

How to use model:

Stimuli frame is the characteristics of the stimuli as perceived by the individual.

Cognitive capacities imply the patient's ability to process information.

Structure providers are the health care providers or support group that can affect the patient either negatively or positively.

Stimuli frame, cognitive capacities, and structure providers are all antecedents to uncertainty. Uncertainty can either be a positive or negative (or a danger or seen as an opportunity).

Inference is how the patients sees themselves as part of the environment and illusion is how they want to be. Either of these can lead to danger making uncertainty a negative experience or to an opportunity as a positive. The use of coping mechanisms can lead to adaptation to the uncertainty of illness.

"The uncertainty theory explains how patients cognitively process illness-related stimuli and construct meaning in these events. Uncertainty, or the inability to structure meaning, can develop if the patient does not form a cognitive schema for illness events" (Mishel, 1988). According to Mishel, the individual moves through distinct processes in experiencing uncertainty:

The beginning of the illness event:

Stimuli Frame: the form in which the patient experiences the initial stimuli

- **Symptom Pattern:** the severity to which a symptom may exist with enough consistency to form a pattern.

Example: chronic cough or unexplained shortness of breath that leads patient to seek treatment

- **Event Familiarity:** repetition and familiarity of the environment.
  ❖ Example: familiar physican/office in contrast to new hospital, staff, new specialists.

- **Event Congruency:** expected events compared to actual illness events.
  ❖ Example: remission versus reoccurrence

Two factors influence the stimuli frame:

Cognitive Capacity: the ability of the individual to process information – this can be impaired by pain, drugs, side effects, fatigue.

Structure Providers: resources available to assist the individual including: Credible Authority: physicians, nurses, staff, Social Support: family, friends, clergy and the level of Education; those with higher education have been shown to process uncertainty more efficiently and effectively than those with less education.

The individual, at this point, experiences some level of uncertainty and so the search for the meaning of the uncertainty begins:

In processing uncertainty, individuals utilize two cognitive processes to achieve appraisal, or the decision of how to perceive uncertainty.

1. Inference: the evaluation of uncertainty is directed by personality strengths and weaknesses, past personal experiences, general knowledge and context.
2. Illusion: development of personal beliefs as a result of the uncertainty experience; these beliefs can include denial or hope, and can be maladaptive or supportive.

The individual then appraises the uncertainty, deciding if the illness event is one of danger or opportunity. (Braden & Mishel, 1988; Mishel, 1988; Neville, 2003)

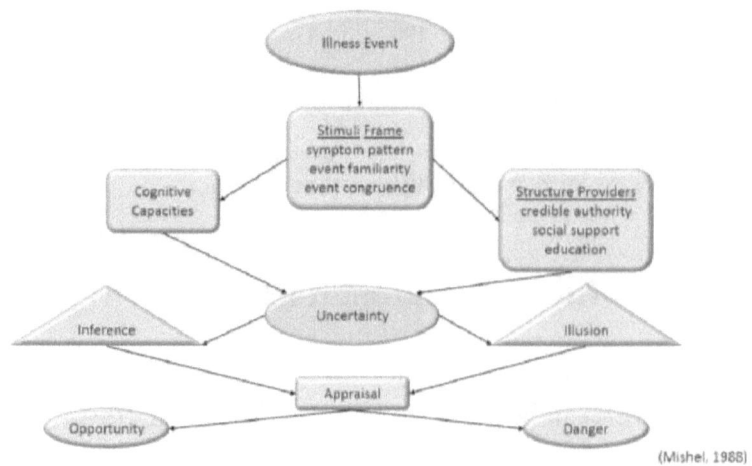

(Mishel, 1988)

"The experience of uncertainty is neutral; it is neither a desired or avoided experience until it is appraised" (Mishel, 1988).

Therefore, uncertainty can be judged by the individual as danger (negative) or opportunity (positive) (Mishel, 1988).

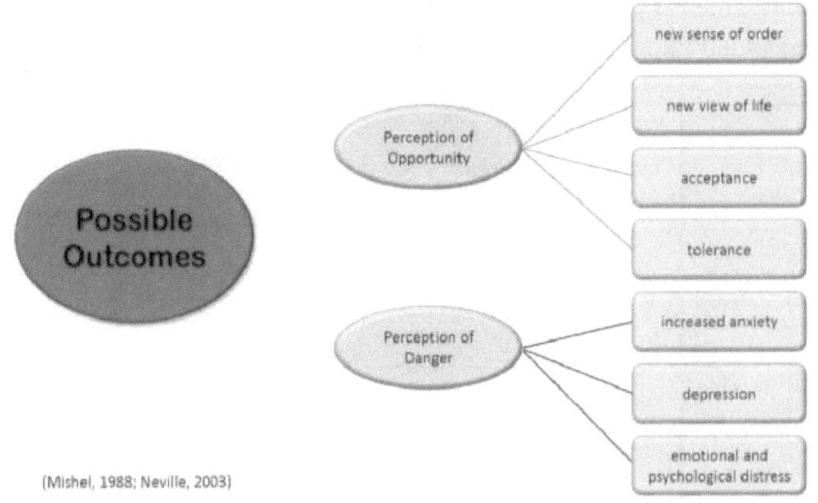

(Mishel, 1988; Neville, 2003)

(Mishel, 1988; Neville, 2008)

THE MISHEL UNCERTAINTY IN ILLNESS SCALE (Community) SAMPLE

Page 1 of 5

ID Number_____

MISHEL UNCERTAINTY IN ILLNESS SCALE (Community) SAMPLE

Do not administer.

INSTRUCTIONS:

Please read each statement. Take your time and think about what each statement says. Then place an "X" under the column that most closely measures how you are feeling TODAY. If you agree with a statement, then you would mark under either "Strongly Agree" or "Agree." If you disagree with a statement, then mark under either "Strongly Disagree" or "Disagree." If you are undecided about how you feel, then mark under "Undecided" for that statement. Please respond to every statement.

	Strongly agree 5	Agree 4	Undecided 3	Disagree 2	Strongly Disagree 1
1 I am unsure of my illness is getting better <u>or worse</u>.					
2 The doctors says things to me that could have many meanings.					
3 It is difficult to know if the treatments or medications I am getting are helping.					
4 Because of the unpredictability of my illness, I cannot plan for the future.					
5 The seriousness of my illness has been determined.					

ID Number_____

MISHEL UNCERTAINTY IN ILLNESS SCALE (Adult) SAMPLE

Do not administer.

INSTRUCTIONS:

Please read each statement. Take your time and think about what each statement says. Then place an "X" under the column that most closely measures how you are feeling TODAY. If you agree with a statement, then you would mark under either "Strongly Agree" or "Agree." If you disagree with a statement, then mark under either "Strongly Disagree" or "Disagree." If you are undecided about how you feel, then mark under "Undecided" for that statement. Please respond to every statement.

	Strongly agree 5	Agree 4	Undecided 3	Disagree 2	Strongly Disagree 1
1 I have a lot of questions without <u>answers</u>.					
2 I understand everything explained to me.					
3 The doctors say things to me that could have many meanings.	ix.				

	Strongly agree 5	Agree 4	Undecided 3	Disagree 2	Strongly Disagree 1
4 There are so many different types of staff, it's unclear who is responsible for what.					
5 The purpose of each treatment is clear to me.					

ID Number_____

MISHEL UNCERTAINTY IN ILLNESS SCALE (Parent/Child) SAMPLE

Do not administer.

INSTRUCTIONS:

Please read each statement. Take your time and think about what each statement says. Then place an "X" under the column that most closely measures how you are feeling TODAY. If you agree with a statement, then you would mark under either "Strongly Agree" or "Agree." If you disagree with a statement, then mark under either "Strongly Disagree" or "Disagree." If you are undecided about how you feel, then mark under "Undecided" for that statement. Please respond to every statement.

	Strongly agree 5	Agree 4	Undecided 3	Disagree 2	Strongly Disagree 1
1 It is unclear how bad my child's pain will be.					
2 I can predict how long my child's illness will last.					
3 Because of the unpre-dictability of my child's illness, I cannot plan for the future.					

Page 5 of 5

	Strongly agree 5	Agree 4	Undecided 3	Disagree 2	Strongly Disagree 1
1 It's vague to me how I will manage the care of my child after he/she leaves the hospital.					
2 I'm certain they will not find anything else wrong with my child.					

CHAPTER 8

ASSESSMENT MODELS AND TOOLS
IN FAMILY MEDICINE

A WIDE ARRAY of tools have been used and adapted for use to assess various aspects of the family. We shall examine some of these tools in this chapter.

GENOGRAM: Family Diagram

A **genogram** is a graphic representation of a family tree that displays detailed data on relationships among individuals. It goes beyond a traditional family tree by allowing the user to analyze hereditary patterns and psychological factors that punctuate relationships. The genogram maps out relationships and traits that may otherwise be missed on a pedigree chart. Genograms were first developed and popularized in clinical settings by Monica McGoldrick and Randy Gerson. Genograms are now used by various groups of people in a variety of fields such as medicine, psychology, social work, genealogy, genetic research, and education. Genograms contain a wealth of information on the families represented. First, they contain basic data found in family trees such as the name, gender, date of birth, and date of death of each individual. Additional data may include education, occupation, major life events, chronic illnesses, social behaviors, nature of family relationships, emotional relationships, and social relationships. Some genograms also include information on disorders running in the family such as alcoholism, depression, diseases, alliances, and living situations. Genograms can vary significantly because there is no limitation as to what type of data can be included.

A genogram is therefore a graphical representation of a person's family relationship and medical history. It is a unique type of family research diagram. It not only records family members and their relationships to each other, but also many of their physical and physiological attributes by utilizing an elaborate system of symbols.

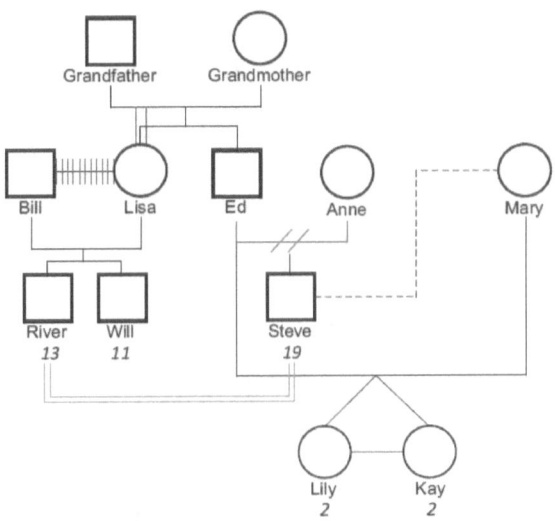

ECOMAP

This is a casual representation of the family unit in relationship to its suprasystems; outside world, community, support systems, etc.

An **eco-map** (or **ecomap**) is a graphical representation that shows all of the systems at play in an individual's life. Eco-maps are used in individual and family counseling They are often a way of portraying Systems Theory in a simplistic way that both the family physician and the patient/client can look at during the session. These ecological maps, or ecomaps, were developed by Hartman in 1975 as a means of depicting the ecological system that encompasses a family or individual (Hartman, 1995). An **ecogram** is a combination of a genogram and an ecomap. The terms "ecogram" and "ecomap" are often used interchangeably,

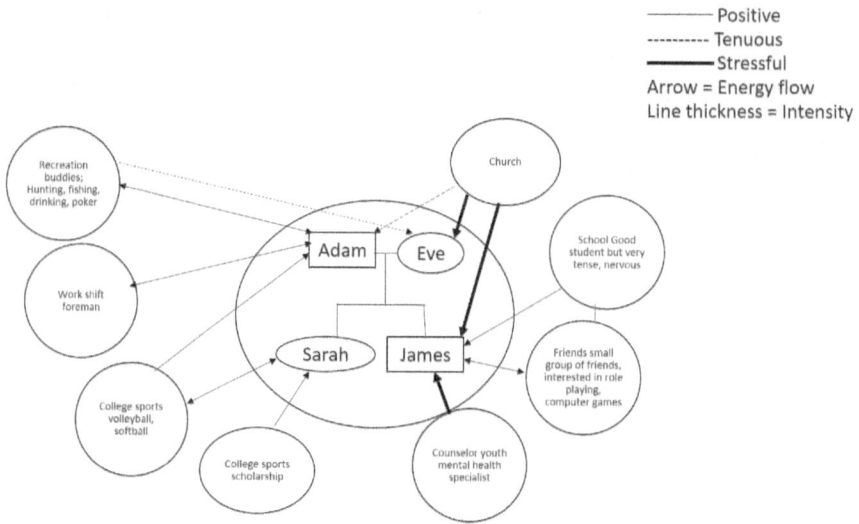

FAMILY CIRCLE AND SOCIOGRAM

The Family Circle is a graphic method for disclosing dynamics of family interaction using circles. In a **Sociogram** person draws circles to indicate significant persons in his or her life.

The family circle can be regarded as a variation of sociogram

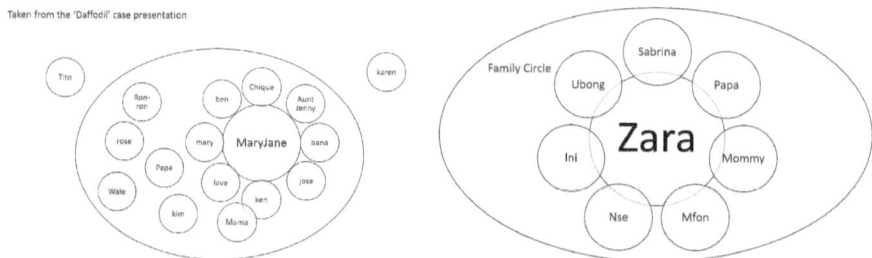

Taken from the 'Daffodil' case presentation

Family Map

Family map was developed by Salvador Minuchin a psychiatrist family therapist in order to facilitate communications of information about a family system to colleagues so that they can be understood.

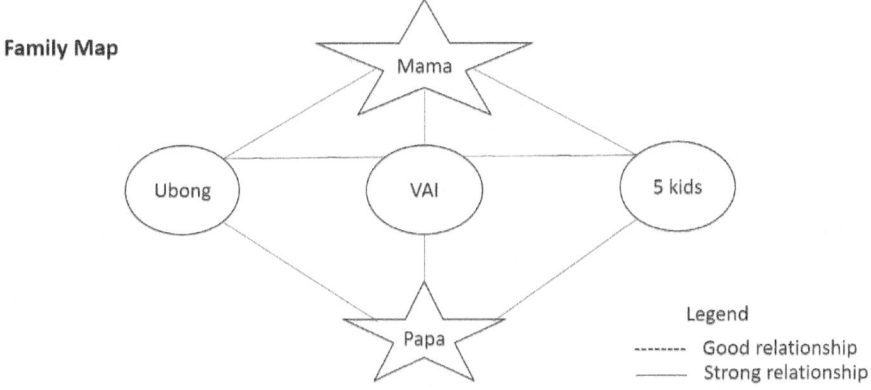

Family Map

Legend

-------- Good relationship
———— Strong relationship

Family APGAR

The family Apgar may be used to determine the level of functionalism in the family unit. This data will assist the family physician in identifying appropriate interventions. It is a screening questionnaire about family member's satisfaction with functional state of the family (see Wong) Rapid screening test instrument for family dysfunction. It has adequate reliability and validity to measure individual's level of satisfaction about family relationship

A – ADAPTATION
P – PARTNERSHIP
G – GROWTH
A – AFFECTION
R – RESOLVE

When is a Family APGAR really needed?

1. When a family is directly involved in the care the patient.
2. When treating a new patient in order to serve as a general view of family function.
3. When treating a patient whose family is in crisis.
4. When a patients behavior makes the family physician suspect a psychosocial problem possibly due to family dysfunction.

THE FAMILY APGAR QUESTIONNAIRE

Introduction: The following questions have been designed to help us better understand you and your family. You should feel free to ask questions about any item in the questionnaire. Answer each question as "almost always", "sometimes", or "hardly ever". Add any additional comments you want. Family is defined as the individual(s) with whom you usually live.

For each question, check only one box.

Almost always Some of the time **Hardly ever**

1. I am satisfied that I can turn to my family for help when something is troubling me.

Comments:

2. I am satisfied that my family talks things over. With me and shares problems with me.

Comments:

3. I am satisfied that my family accepts and supports my wishes to take on new activities or directions

Comments:_____

4. I am satisfied that my family expresses affection and responds to my emotions, such as anger, sorrow and love.

Comments:_____

5. I am satisfied with the way my family and I share time together.

Comments:_____

Scoring: The patient checks one of three choices which are scored as follows: "Almost always" (2 points), "Some of the time" (1 point), or "Hardly ever) (0 points). The scores for each of the five questions are then totaled.

A score of 7-10 suggests a highly functional family. A score of 4 to 6 suggests a moderately dysfunctional family. A score of 0 to 3 suggests a severely dysfunctional family.

According to which member of the family is being interviewed the family doctor my substitute for the word "family" either spouse, significant other, parents or children. (Smilkstein 1978).

SCREEM tool

Is Important for the assessment of the family capacity to participate in the provision of health care and coping with crisis. The forces which affect the family have been described by Smilkstein and summarized by his acronym SCREEM;

Social: including factors such as medical care, leisure time, resources, and community networks and organizations that impact most immediately on the patient.

Cultural: including religious factors which are closely related to ethnic and racial background.

Economic: including level of **Education** and type and level of **Employment**; all three 'Es' being closely intertwined.

Medical-Political: including legal and policy decisions, usually originating at the national level.

Home Observation for Management of the Environment (HOME) tool

This is used in the home to assess a child's environment, different inventories for different age groups, some items based on observation, others on questions to parents.

Home Screening Questionnaire (HSQ)

Based on the HOME but is a questionnaire that can be completed by the parents in any setting.

Tools which require family drawings:

Sociogram person draws circles to indicate significant persons in his or her life.

Family circle variation of sociogram.

Kinetic family drawing (KFD) person draw the family "doing something".

Conjoint family drawing family draw it together, focus.

CHAPTER 9

THE PRACTICE OF FAMILY MEDICINE

Family Practice Model: Reason for Encounter

THE LACK OF a distinctive model for family medicine in West Africa hampers the progress of the discipline several was. For example, as family physicians we are using different models, it is understandable that morbidity studies in the discipline are often at great variance with one another, this tend to bring conflict during examinations when candidates feel a disconnect from the examiner in the interpretation of a patient's symptom in order to come to a diagnosis. Does the candidate interpret his encounter with the patient solely in the traditional biomedical paradigm or in the biopsychosocial context? Furthermore, in the teaching of the discipline, the absence of a definitive commonly agreed model by the faculty makes the learning, teaching and evaluation extremely difficult and the wide variation of trainer's models make the exercise highly subjective. The line of least resistance is to resort to the Newtonian model to explain our method. However, the most important objective of any interaction and therefore the crux of our clinical competence are to establish the reasons for the patient's attendance (RFE-reason for encounter) – the components of his illness. In the short time available, attention must be paid to detail of the patient's presentation, since all that he says and does and does not, in this concentrated time (which has perhaps followed days or even years of indecision), must surely be relevant. The reason for his attendance can be expressed in terms of his "feelings and fears", his "ideas", how his "functioning" has been affected and his "expectations" (FIFE). This the family physician factors into the management of the patient.

It is quite clear that this contention does not invalidate the contribution made by disease or doctor-centered medicine but merely attempts to explain the family physician's perspective of medicine in the understanding and management of illness. Therefore, an obvious way out is to sufficiently weave all models into training, examination and research so as to have relevance to Family Medicine in West Africa.

General Comments

Every interaction between a conscious patient and a doctor involves a consultation of one form of another. The nature of that consultation and the manner in which it is conducted could influence the outcome of that interaction considerably. It could influence the doctor's understanding of the patient's condition; the patient's reaction to the condition and his ability to cope; compliance; the satisfaction of the patient or the doctor; and even the patient's life.

When a patient seeks a doctor's help the doctor must endeavour to discover the patients reason for encounter; make an hypothesis based on what the patient says or demonstrates, and what the doctor is able to find on examination; test out the hypothesis, make as final assessment as possible, explain what he has found, administer appropriate management, which may include medication; and concluding that particular consultation by giving advise to the patient about how to take things further. At the same time, the doctor should attempt to develop an ongoing relationship with that patient to enhance and encourage continuity of care.

Unfortunately when we were medical students very rarely get the opportunity to experience this 'total care' of a patient who seeks their specific assistance, unless they work at a community clinic or in a similar situation. Their usual training in this regard is limited to a segment of the consultation (even if an important one), i.e. extracting a history of a complaint, and examining a 'case' and then presenting the findings related to the disease to the teacher. It is unfortunate that the student very rarely has the opportunity to practice the art of 'caring' for a person, from the initial help-seeking, through the assessment to the management and 'goodbye', even with simulated patients!

Episodes and Encounters

Components of PHC Encounter

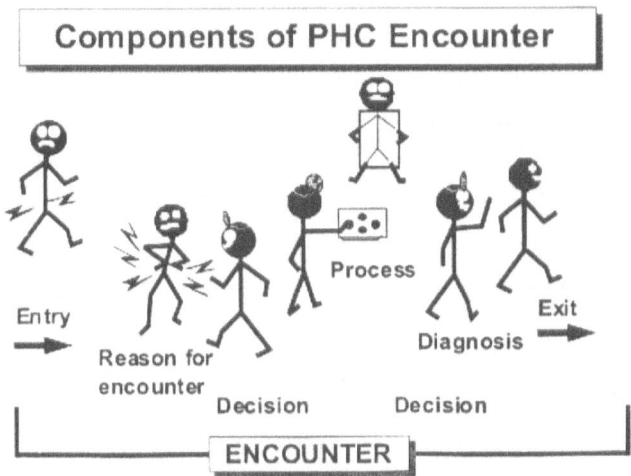

Components of the Encounter in an episode of illness.

Lamberts & Wood

Lamberts, Wood and others have been instrumental in developing an International Classification for Primary Care (ICPC) which is used extensively for the classification of the work done by family practitioners. The ICD9 and ICD10 systems of WHO are of little value in classifying the many facets in an episode of illness. An episode of disease is defined as a problem or illness in a patient over the entire period of time from its onset to its resolution. Using this definition an episode of illness can be expected to include several encounters, (single consultations) such as that illustrated above.

The ICPC can be used to classify all the phases - reason for encounter, initial diagnosis, any processes undertaken (tests, procedures etc.) to establish a more definite diagnosis, followup processes (drugs, operations etc.) and outcomes such as referrals etc. A patient could 'exit' to his home, to another doctor or agency, to hospital, and also 'exit' to return for another encounter related to a particular episode of illness.

More recently, WONCA (The World Organisation of Family Practitioners) developed COOP Charts which are able to classify the functional status of the patient, adding to a more complete understanding of the *patient*, the *disease*, his *illness* and the *sickness*.

The biopsychosocial model is a philosophy of clinical care and a practical clinical guide. Philosophically, it is a way of understanding how suffering, disease, and illness are affected by multiple levels of organization, from the social to the subatomic particle using the General System Theory. A major hindrance in the advancement of family practice in West Africa as a discipline is the insistence on describing it in the terminology of traditional biomedical medicine. The traditional biomedical medicine, the doctor fits the patient's illness into a precise class linking the symptoms and signs with organic pathology and identifying single external causes. He explains the patient's illness in terms of his own worldview during the consultative process by taking a domineering stance on the assumption that he, the doctor has sufficient knowledge and skills about the positive health outcome of the individual patient. On the other hand, family Medicine interprets symptoms in terms of its own method and objectives. Interpretation of the patient (patient-centered method) rather than the symptoms (disease-centered method) is the crux of clinical competence in family practice. This method is consistent with Einsteinium in physics rather than Newtonian physics which are the basis of traditional biomedical medicine. The value of the biosychosocial model is not the discovery of a new scientific law, but the application of medical knowledge the needs of each patient for which the family physician is adequately trained. This forms the basic science background for the training of family physician in West Africa as envisaged by the founding fathers in 1980s.

The scientific basis of Family Medicine in West Africa which sometimes appears woolly and rooted as an art-cum-science form continues to be a positive dilemma leading to incisive discussions as to whether family medicine is a distinct clinical specialty in its own right or collectively putting together portions of care from other major clinical specialty or a subspecialty of community health. Specialties are considered to arise from a primordial stem of basic medical training in the Flexnerian style leading to a reduction study in a core clinical area while family medicine thrives in the generalist genre. Therefore what constitute the domain, context and contextual paradigm for the practice of family medicine are depicted in the 3 concentric circles.

Family Medicine Practice consists of 3 Core Areas

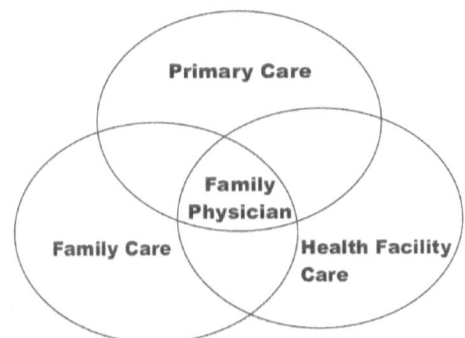

Family Medicine Practice consists of 3 Core Areas

Primary Care consists of two areas of care, primary medical care and primary health care.

Primary Care consists of two areas of care, primary medical care and primary health care.

Primary Medical Care

The term primary care was first used in 1920 in Britain to distinguish health care given in clinical and general practices from secondary care delivered in hospitals. The term was later expanded to include primary medical or clinical care. Primary care is used to refer to all care delivered at the first or primary level in contrast with care delivered in the hospital. Throughout the world, general practitioners/family physicians deliver most medical care at the primary level. In their work, they assume responsibility for the patient, beginning at the time of the first encounter and continuing thereafter. This includes overall management and coordination of health care, such as the appropriate use of specialist care and other health care resources. In Nigeria, the people have relied on private medical practitioners to ensure that primary care is made universally accessible. Issues of travel, sport medicine, men's, adolescent, reproductive, first line geriatric and occupational health are managed at this level.

Table 9.1

THE 5 STAR ROLE OF THE FAMILY PHYSICIAN IN PRIMARY MEDICAL CARE

CARE PROVIDER	Who considers the patients as an integral part of a family and the community and provides high standard clinical care. Manages chronic disease and disability and personalizes preventive care with a long-term trusting relationship.
DECISION MAKER	Who choose which technologies to apply ethically and cost-effectively while enhancing the care that he or she provides

COMMUNICATOR	Who is able to promote healthy lifestyles by emphatic explanation, thereby empowering the individual and groups to enhance and protect their health.
ADVOCATE/ COMMUNITY LEADER	Who having won the trust of the people among whom he or she works can reconcile individual and community health requirements and initiate action on behalf of the community.
MANAGER/TEAM MEMBER,	Who can work harmoniously with individuals and organizations, within and without the health care system to meet the patient's and community's needs.

Primary Health Care (PHC)

The World Health Organization (1978) defined primary health care as essential health care made universally accessible to individuals and families in the community by means acceptable to them, through their full participation and at a cost that the community and the country can afford. It forms an integral part of the countries health system. Primary health care system, is the nucleus, and of the overall socio-economic development of the community.' Primary health care. In its broadest sense is a philosophy or set of values and principles for organizing the health system as a whole. The acquisition of skills for community participation form the cornerstone of the leadership role expected of the family physician.

Table 9.2 Roles of the Family physician in Primary Health Care

ADVOCACY	Family Physicians are expected to be advocates of health to policy makers. This is due to the strategic position they play in health care. Consequent to this is their ability to mobilize the family and community effectively for health actions. Of course it is expected that they have a firm grasp of community diagnosis through baseline information and updated situation analysis of their community.
TRAINING	Family physicians are expected to be involved in the training of the other cadre of health care personnel whether in the hospital as medical students, nurses, nursing aides, auxiliaries or in the community as volunteer health worker (VHWs) Community health extension worker (CHEWs) and community health officers (CHOs)
SUPERVISION	The family physician as a leader of the primary and secondary health care teams has to have skills to supervise the activities to those working with him. It is given that such supervision is appropriate and arises from the fact that as a well trained family physician he is delegating his roles and therefore can assume them when need be.
RESEARCH	Family physicians have to give leadership in practice based research networks. It is expected that they are able to develop protocols, and mobilize private practitioners and other primary care practitioners find answers to basic conditions that present to them before they require hospital management.
MONITORING AND EVALUATION	Is an expected skill arising firm above roles

Family Dynamics and Family Care

Central to the practice of Family Medicine is the understanding of the concept of what the family is, the dynamics of its processes and the components of its care.

The family has a great impact on the rehabilitation of chronic disease patients and terminal care. It influences the causation of acute disease. It determines therapeutic success or failure (including medication compliance). It determines the degree of mental health and illness and plays a major role in preventive and wellness aspects of health care (through culture, beliefs, practices and spirituality).

The Family is defined as a social and intimate nurturing group of individuals connected to a patient biologically, legally, or by choice, from whom the patient can reasonably expect a measure of support in the form of food, shelter, finance and emotional nurturing; that shares a past, a present and a future with the patient and includes all who contribute in one way or the other to the family culture.

Hospital and Clinic Care

In West Africa, the family physician functions as a general, community physician, surgeon, obstetrician and gynecologist especially in the private rural/ practice and as community physician in the government. The expectations of them are very high and a superior level of clinical competence is assumed.

The focus of the residency training has been concentrated in this area for the obvious reason that many of the skills required could best be accessed in the hospital environment.

Unfortunately this has led to the confusion that residents are being trained as composite mini-specialist. It has also made colleagues in other specialties especially the major specialty to feel that a hostile takeover is in the offing. Actually major aspects of training tale place in areas likes the General outpatient Departments, Accident and Emergency (NHIS) Departments where frontline medicine is practiced.

CHAPTER 10

THE FAMILY PHYSICIAN

FAMILY MEDICINE AS a discipline has been informed by general systems theory, which was developed in response to the limitations of nineteenth- century science and of the biomedical approach. The systems theory has provided the basis for the biopsychosocial model of illness. These concepts have been discussed in greater detail during the block. The principles which underpin the discipline and govern our actions have been admirably expounded by Professor Ian McWhinney of London, Western Ontario. None of them is unique to Family Medicine and not all family doctors exemplify all nine. In his words; 'Nevertheless, when taken together, they do represent a distinctive world view – a system of values and an approach to problems – that is identifiably different from that of other disciplines.' The principles can be summarized as follows:

Summary of McWhinney's Principles

1. The family physician is **committed to the person** rather than to a particular body of knowledge, group of diseases, or special technique.
2. The family physician seeks to understand the **context** of the illness.
3. The family physician sees every contact with his patients as an **opportunity for prevention** or health education.
4. The family physician views his practice as a **population at risk.**
5. The family physician sees himself as part of a communitywide **network** of supportive and health care agencies.
6. Ideally the family physician should share the **same habitat** as his patients.

7. The family physician sees patients at the **office (rooms), at their homes, and in hospital.**
8. The family physician attaches importance to the **subjective aspects** of medicine.
9. The family physician is a **manager of resources.**

Implications of the Principles

The implications of the above principles on the practice of Family Medicine are numerous. The nature of a family doctor's commitment to patients requires him to provide continuing and comprehensive care. These include but are not limited to the following:

Continuity of Care

Continuity of care becomes a responsibility and a commitment by the practitioner. It is one of the hallmarks of family practice. It is a commitment despite referral, death, failure or cure, and whether the patient is seeking health care or not.

Comprehensiveness of Care

Since family practitioners are available for any type of health problem, irrespective of the age or sex of the patient, or which organ or system is affected, the care they provide is comprehensive. Even referral does not imply that the irresponsibility has ended.

Bonding

Strong bonds can develop between the doctor and his/her patients, depending on the duration and intensity of care. Such bonding can have major implications on patient and doctor satisfaction. It is particularly strengthened by certain types of care such as caring for a patient during pregnancy and childbirth, at times of crisis, and terminal care.

Cumulative Knowledge of Patients

Continuous and comprehensive care allows a family practitioner to gather extensive knowledge over time about the patients and families in his/her care. Such knowledge is extremely valuable in understanding and caring for patients.

Are we training or trained for it?

The faculty of General Medical Practice has changed its name to the Faculty of Family Medicine. The change has come partly due to worldwide response to the call by the world organization of family doctors calling on all colleges, academies, societies and associations of general practitioners that have a postgraduate/specialty program to change and due to pressure from societal view of the certified members not being regarded as a specialist. Also the public view of not being able to differentiate those with a basic medical degree from those who have acquired specialist qualification from the general practitioners has prompted this paper. Using a convenient sample of key informants who were faculty officers in the national postgraduate medical college of Nigeria and the west African college of physicians faculty of general medical practice/family practice who sourced information from documents and the internet the extent to which family doctors are being trained to be relevant in the west African subregion was explored.

The principles, attributes and skills for family practice in a developing economy as ours is highlighted. It is the breath of care of family practice with a depth of competencies that makes the difference from general medical practice.

The concept of the family as an interacting system with its own particular problems of maintenance and action is changing. Therefore it has to be determined whether the idea of the family as a unit of service or valid on the Nigeria health scene. Each family can be regarded as a unique small-scale community with its own internal organization and world view.

For a family physician the insights of medical anthropologists and psychologist are useful in understanding the role of the family in health, illness and medical care. What the ICCR has recommended is that the individual and the family should become the key focus of family medicine in Nigeria. How many practitioners see the family itself as a collective patient with its own specific health problems? Do GPs have the mandate of the individual to manage him in the context of other family members?

Globally, we have common concerns on the skills, attitudes and knowledge necessary to be a good family physician. However, special problems about family medicine in the context of medical care in relation to primary health care continue to haunt the faculty. This is as a result of paradigm shift on the track of medicine from a biomedical model focused on the management of acute diseases in hospital to a biopsychosocial model on the management of acute, chronic and preventive illnesses in the community.

The essence of general practice is being on the right point on that track at the right time and having the skills to work effectively there. The family physician is classed as a generalist. This group includes primary care physicians, general practitioners and family physicians. In Nigeria, the generalist often functions as a five star doctor, as a general physician and surgeon in private practice and a community physician, obstetrician gynaecologist and surgeon when in government service in the rural area. The expectations of them are very high and a superior level of clinical competence is assumed.

This paper intends to give a contextual and conceptual view of this change, and is directed at the problem of the training of a family physician in Nigeria by answering the following questions about the general practitioner (GP) and family physician (FP)

1. Who is a family physician in Nigeria?
2. In what way is family physician involved in continuing care?

3. Are family physician members of the primary health care team?
4. What is their understanding of the health team?

The WONCA definition clearly gives an insight to that expectation viz: The GP or FP is the physician who is primarily responsible for providing comprehensive health care to every individual seeking medical care and arranging for other health personnel to provide services when necessary. The GP/FP functions as a generalist and accepts everyone seeking care whereas other health providers limit access to their services on the basis of age, sex and/or diagnosis.

The GP/FP cares for the individual in the context of the family and the family in the context of the community irrespective of race, religion, culture or social class. He is clinically competent to provide the greater part of their care after taking into account their cultural, socio-economical and psychological background. In addition he takes personal responsibility for providing comprehensive and continuing care for his patients. The definition proffered at the 1980 of GPs in Nigeria was very direct in concentrating on the level of care, but although it did not specifically mention the family but still addressed the comprehensiveness of the care to be provided. A general practitioner was defined as a frontline medical practitioner or doctor of first contact who delivers comprehensive health care either privately or in public service.

These definitions place squarely the responsibility on the family physician to provide primary medical care as well as primary health care (PHC). For example the family physician may not be in a position to provide water and sanitation services a component of PHC, but can definitely assist in health educational and promotional activates to prevent cholera or guinea worm infections. The family fits well in the work schedule of the family physician., for in working, his diagnosis objectives are broad, in which case he has to take into account the psychological and social aspect as well as the physical.

Conceptual Issues

The mandate offered by a person consulting the GP cannot be assumed to include other members of his family. To consider the family as the unit of care, requires the GP to look the individual and study the family dynamics as part of the causation of illness in the person.

From the family medicine perspective, the family can be considered as a mini society based on social, psychological and biological criteria and one which mediates between the individual and the wider community or society. Many of Nigerians continue to live in and believe in the importance of a family or a family or a family like-structure.

The majority of Nigerians lives in nuclear or extended families and maintains traditional family roles with the father as the primary bread winner and the mother as the socializer and home manager. While it is likely that this traditional family structure will prevail for some time to come, there are already visible changes such as labour saving equipment, changes from the traditional diet to quick fix proceeded and refined food, early school admission and public recreational facilities have reduced the home making time. There is also growing involvement of women in the labour force with the husband and wife pursuing their career separately.

The family as a group generates, prevents, tolerates or corrects health problems within its membership. Health problems may be caused by many factors such as genetic faults like as sickle cell disease (SCD), alcoholic, behavioral irregularities or catastrophic illness. Disease can be transmitted from parent to child HIV/AIDS. Prolonged stress in the family may cause emotional illness that result in divorce. Conversely the skills and confidence of family functioning together not only facilitates treatment and provides physical support but also lends emotional strength to an afflicted member. The health problems of families are interlocking. The child with a developmental disability (cerebral palsy) may affect the health of his siblings because he requires more parental time and energy. What happens to one member of the family has some affect upon the family collectively and requires the accommodation on the part of one family member. If the mother is ill for example the survival of the children may be jeopardized.

The family is the most frequent source of decision making about health and personal care. Care for minor illness, long- term illness, or disability and pr-hospital and family members generally provide post hospital care during acute illness at home. It is most often the family unit not the individual or the health professionals that decides whether the individual should seek or use health care or not. The family unit is an effective and available channel in which family physician can function, as it becomes the members whom he cannot personally see. By working with the family unit, the family physician is likely to fulfill his obligation to reach the entire community.

Contextual Issues

The family does not exist in vacuum as there are issues that are external to the family, Members, are influenced by a number of factors including economic status culture, religion, ethnicity, locality and residence. Origin personal and family idiosyncrasies as well as wider social, historical and economic forces also exert their influences Factors such as poverty or unemployment may either strengthen or weaken the family. Faces with economic deprivation some families may form tightly knit communities for mutual support while other may quickly disintegrate.

Some of the questions, which should be raised by the family physician to obtain an adequate family history, include the following:

a) How many are there in the family?
b) Who lives at home?
c) In what phase of the family life cycle is the family?
d) What problem does this raise for them?

e) What major problem has the family had in the past e.g. death, separation, divorce, financial crisis, major illness?
f) How is major decision in the family taken?
g) What are the education level and financial status of members?
h) Who are the friends in the neighborhood, including clubs and social societies?
i) Are in-law and relations helpful or do they create problems?

These are the kinds of questions, which would be expected to be asked by residents training in General Practice during their clinical Part One examinations. However of the 12 candidates (examined at the part one level in the two years preceding the writing of the original version of this paper) who had patients with non-communicable diseases such as diabetes, hypertension and sickle cell disease, none took a history concerning the family and effect of the ill health on other members of the household. Residents should be taught these skills in an integrated fashion by their preceptors during training.

Conclusion

The constant and important socio-economic and political change, in the West Africa that the Faculty of General Practice adapts and proactively contributes to the improvement of equity and quality health care, producing Family Physicians who are responsible to social and societal needs, competent not only with scientific knowledge, technical skills and managerial capability but also with the ability to work within the existing model of health care system required to be trained. He should be prepared to reach out to the least privileged in society. From the above have we really trained our residents in biopsychosocio-anthropological milieu to warrant them referred to as family physicians? The present training has not emphasized these functions nor explored the family dynamics in the management of the patient in the context of the family. This is an area, which must seriously be considered before we lose our unique medical model which has been exported to other third world countries.

Principles Underpinning the Practice of Family Medicine

1. Commitment to the person rather than to particular body knowledge, group of diseases, or special technique.
2. Not limited by the type of health problem, sex and age.
3. No define end point of care.
4. Seek to understand the context of the illness. To understand a thing rightly, we need to see it both out of its environment and in it and to have acquaintance with the whole range of its variation" 'William James.
5. Sees every contact with patients as an opportunity for prevention or health education.
6. View his or her practice as a population at risk.
7. Sees himself or herself as part of a community wide network of supportive and health care agencies.
8. Ideally, share the same habitat as their parents.
9. Sees patients at the office, in their homes and in the hospital
10. Attaches importance to the subjective aspect of medicine
11. Awareness of self understands that their own values attitude and feeling are important determinants of how they practice medicine.
12. Manages resources
13. Control of admission to hospital
14. Use of investigations
15. Prescription of treatment Referral to specialist

Essential Attributes of Family Physicians

1. Take an approach to health care which puts into practice the principles of system theory, which express the interrelatedness of biological, psychology, family, occupational social, economic, community and environmental factor in health and illness.

2. Exhibit clinical competence over a wide range of patient problems and provide comprehensive care.
3. Take a person centered approach. Which build up a trusting doctor patient relationship?
4. Provide this personal care in the context of home. Work place and community.
5. Provide continuity of care context of home, work place and community.
6. Provide continuity of care over long period.
7. Have an orientation to the family and the home. Influence on health and illness.
8. Have an awareness of the workplace and the community, and the health issues there.
9. Maintain a consistent focus on anticipatory care prevention and health promotion at a personal, family and community level.
10. Care for defined practice population.
11. Have knowledge of health care resources of the community.
12. Arrange appropriate referral to other health resources, and shared care where appropriate.
13. Provide cost-effective and efficient health care in a community setting.
14. Undertaking quality assessment of their practice and continuing education to remedy deficiencies.
15. Carry out research into the fundamentals of family medicine. These attributes encapsulate the dominant unchanging values of family practice.

In conclusion, the principles, attributes and skills for family practice in a developing economy as ours is that of a doctor with integrated comprehensive care that is far superior to that attained from basic medical education or the focused and narrow specialist course. It is the breath of care of family practice with a depth of competencies that makes the difference.

VICTOR INEM

COMMUNICATION IN PRACTICE BAD NEWS

Bad news can be defined as any information that drastically alters a patient's view of the future for the worse (Baile et al 2000).

S - Setting up the interview
P - Patients **Perceptions**
I - Invitation to ascertain how much the person wants to know
K - Knowledge and information giving
E - Emotion management
S - Strategy and **Summary** of the key points

A patient has a right but not a duty to hear bad news.

Most patients want two things:

1. A certain amount of information (the right amount)
2. The opportunity to talk and think about their situation (ie. a therapeutic dialogue).

Breaking bad news is important to maintain trust between the patient and doctor, to reduce uncertainty, to prevent inappropriate hope, to allow appropriate adjustment, and to prevent a conspiracy of silence that destroys family communication and prevents mutual support.

Breaking bad news can be broadly broken down into six steps.

1. Preparation
2. Ask questions to start the negotiation.
3. Explain in steps.
4. Elicit concerns and feelings.
5. Summarize
6. Offer availability and follow up.

1. **Preparation**

   a) Know all the facts, i.e. what has happened before and what the management options are.

   b) Who should be present; It is often best for a doctor and nurse to see the patient and relative together. The patient should be given the opportunity to have a relative present as they may be in a state of shock.

   c) Set time aside and avoid interruptions and always sit down.

2. **Ask questions**

It is important to hear the patient's narrative of events to allow them to explain what has happened and where they are up to in their illness e.g. Ask "How did it all start?" and "What happened next?" A useful question can be "What has been the most difficult part of the whole thing for you?" This way you understand the patient's perspective and what they understand by their illness and therefore can avoid giving shocking information, if, for example, it is their belief they have had curative treatment when you know that their prognosis is only weeks. There is good evidence that most doctors interrupt the patient within 30 seconds of speaking.

3. **Explain if requested**

For example, ask "Do you want me to go over anything?" The aim is to narrow the information gap. The skill is finding the optimum level of information to reduce uncertainty without causing fear by giving excessive information.

- Be clear and simple.
- Use kind words.
- Give a narrative of events guided by the patient's earlier narrative of events using the same language.

- Avoid medical jargon.
- Check understanding ("Is this making sense?" "Have I covered what you want to talk about?").
- Be as optimistic as possible.
- Deal with concerns before explaining details.

Denial is a way of coping with fear and it should be respected as a coping strategy, especially if the patient is coping. If the patient declines further information, it should be acknowledged, but also acknowledge the discomfort of uncertainty and give permission to ask questions at a later date. Few patients adopt a stance of denial permanently, most start to ask for more information once they feel more secure. Patients usually experience belief once they are able to discuss some of their fears.

4. **Elicit concerns and feelings**

After explaining bad news eliciting concerns is essential. Ask "What is worrying you the most?" Many patients are distressed but can be uncertain what the distress is mainly about. Giving permission to discuss concerns enables the patient to start clarifying the issues and then prioritizing their concerns. This feels like a positive process to the patient and is always helpful. Avoid premature reassurance or excessive explanations, which can cause dissatisfaction and frustration.

Allowing ventilation of feelings provides a therapeutic part of the dialogue. 'How does this leave you feeling at the moment?' is the key phrase. The aim is to help the patient try to name their feelings. Encouraging the ventilation of feelings conveys empathy. Empathy means trying to understand what the patient is feeling, which is much more therapeutic than sympathy (feeling sorry). Our own discomfort during this stage can have an impact on the therapeutic process especially if powerful feelings emerge such as fear, anger. Stay calm and allow time for the person to think about their feelings.

5. **Summarize**

Summarizing is a useful process for patient and doctor. It is supportive and reduces the patient's feeling of confusion at a time of crisis. Making a plan involves a lot of thought and has to integrate the patient's main concerns with the doctor's knowledge of the management options available. It also acknowledges the support system already available to the patient, especially friends and relatives. It helps to explain that it is possible and important to simultaneously prepare for the worst and still hope for the best.

6. **Offer availability**

Follow up is important for three reasons:

a) The details of the information are not remembered at first, rather the way the information was given.
b) Emotional adjustment takes time.
c) It is an opportunity to see other family members/supporters.

Conclusion

It is not always easy to remember the six steps when breaking bad news to a patient. However the principles essentially follow two unbreakable rules when breaking bad news.

1. Ask questions first – What is known? What is wanted? Should relatives be involved?
2. Elicit concerns and encourage the ventilation of feelings.

If you do this you will help your patients and not do any harm.

The above article was based on "Breaking Bad News (Pocket Book)" by Peter Kaye, EPL Publications. The book is extremely useful as a teaching aide and is not available from bookshops. It is available from EPL Publications, 41

Park Avenue North, NorthamptonNN3 2HTUK. Any queries/comments to Joanne Doran.

A FRAMEWORK FOR BREAKING BAD NEWS

Preparation, Beginning the session/setting the scene, Sharing the information, Being sensitive to the patient, Planning and support Follow up and closing References.

Preparation:

- set up appointment as soon as possible
- allow enough uninterrupted time; if seen in surgery, ensure no interruptions
- use a comfortable, familiar environment • invite spouse, relative, friend, as appropriate
- be adequately prepared re clinical situation, records, patient's background
- doctor to put aside own "baggage" and personal feelings wherever possible.

Beginning the session/setting the scene

- Summarize where things have got to date, check with the patient
- discover what has happened since last seen • calibrate how the patient is thinking/feeling
- negotiate agenda.

Sharing the information

- assess the patient's understanding first: what the patient already knows, is thinking or has been told
- gauge how much the patient wishes to know

- give warning first that difficult information coming e.g. "I'm afraid we have some work to do...." "I'm afraid it looks more serious than we had hoped...."
- give basic information, simply and honestly; repeat important points
- relate your explanation to the patient's framework
- do not give too much information too early; don't pussyfoot but do not overwhelm
- give information in small "chunks"; categorise information giving
- watch the pace, check repeatedly for understanding and feelings as you proceed
- use language carefully with regard given to the patient's intelligence, reactions, emotions: avoid jargon.

Being sensitive to the patient

- read the non-verbal clues; face/body language, silences, tears
- allow for "shut down" (when patient turns off and stops listening) and then give time and space: allow possible denial
- keep pausing to give patient opportunity to ask questions
- gauge patient's need for further information as you go and give more information as requested, i.e. listen to the patient's wishes as patients vary greatly in their needs
- encourage expression of feelings, give early permission for them to be expressed: i.e. "how does that news leave you feeling", "I'm sorry that was difficult for you", "you seem upset by that"
- respond to patient's feelings and predicament with acceptance, empathy and concern
- check patient's previous knowledge about information given
- specifically elicit all the patient's concerns
- check understanding of information given ("would you like to run through what are you going to tell your wife?")

- be aware of unshared meanings (i.e. what cancer means for the patient compared with what it means for the physician)
- do not be afraid to show emotion or distress.

Planning and support

- having identified all the patient's specific concerns, offer specific help by breaking down overwhelming feelings into manageable concerns, prioritizing and distinguishing the fixable from the unfixable
- identify a plan for what is to happen next
- give a broad time frame for what may lie ahead
- give hope tempered with realism ("preparing for the worst and hoping for the best")
- ally yourself with the patient ("we can work on this together ...between us") i.e. co-partnership with the patient / advocate of the patient
- emphasize the quality of life
- safety net Follow up and closing
- summarize and check with patient
- don't rush the patient to treatment
- set up early further appointment, offer telephone calls etc.
- identify support systems; involve relatives and friends
- offer to see/tell spouse or others
- make written materials available

Remember doctor's anxiety while giving information, from previous experience, failure to cure or help.

CHAPTER 11

RESEARCH IN PRACTICE WHY FAMILY PRACTICE RESEARCH IS IMPORTANT

F EW PEOPLE WOULD argue that family practice research is not important. Nevertheless it is worth setting out the reasons.

Research improves patient care

This is as true for family practice as any other discipline. In addition to research on primary care illnesses and their management, family practice has some specific needs. It has a high degree of contextual complexity (broad range of relative underdeveloped signs and symptoms, presently within the patient's individual and social setting) compare with the technique complexity of the special (narrow range of defined symptoms across single organ systems, more severe mortality and limited reference to the patient's social context).

The detection of the earliest departure from normal is difficult. High quality family practice research answers questions such as why patients with the same symptoms do, or do not, present to their family practitioner, improve practitioners diagnostic capabilities; understand the natural progression of disease; provide evidence for interventions; and increase understanding of patient compliance. There are gaps in the evidence that clinicians need in making decisions. This limits the provision of the highest quality care in Family practice.

There are several types.
Basic science
Effectiveness (Both effectiveness and cost-effectiveness)

Applicability: Translating evidence generated in non-primary care settings into family practice.

Implementation: Applying what is effective in ideal research conditions into routine family practice.

Research is the main way for teachers to contribute to their discipline

We start from the following premise. Good teachers contribute to the body of knowledge they team Research is the main avenue for this contribution Good research does not guarantee good teaching skills. However the best teachers are intimately involved in the body of knowledge they teach. Teachers of family practice are under-represented by excellence in research (however they over-represent experts in teaching – pedagogy) accordingly they Community-based discipline it is important. Splitting the teaching faculty splits their critical intellectual mass.

Research Stimulates Intellectual Rigor and Critical Thinking

Family practice has a reputation for being among the least intellectually rigorous clinical disciplines. This may have several serious consequences:

a. loss of self-confidence
b. lack of attractiveness as an intellectual area
c. less application of critical thinking in routine clinical work.

Where does research fit with the other clinical duties in family practice?

The predominant responsibilities of family practitioners can be listed as:

Clinical
Administrative
Educative
Research

There are limited empirical data to quantify the breakdown of time allocated by family practitioners to these various tasks. What is an appropriate proportional allocation to these various tasks? Presumably this should vary between different individuals but by what factor? What is ideal? To what extent should research be abdicated to academic? Perhaps all family practitioners should apportion some time to engagement in research as users, participants or leaders.

How do family practitioners acquire research skills?

At least lip service is applied to curriculum statements about acquiring research skills in undergraduate and general practice training. For example, Australian general practice registrars are expected to acquire competence in research during training. The Royal Australian College of General Practitioners training handbook's curriculum states that "... registrars are successfully trained to... contribute to the development of the discipline of general practice and of the RACGP through teaching and research in primary healthcare and public health".

This has not translated into practice research skills and achievements contribute little to graduating. Worse, GP registrars undertaking research during their registrar years are penalized because time spent away from clinical activities to undertake research must be added onto the end of their training period: research lengthens training.

The UK has an inverse law educational opportunities for research training are available least to the branch of medicine that needs them the most. In contrast, in other medical disciplines the acquisition of research skills is explicitly declared an essential component of training, and examined: research is mandatory. Registrars cannot graduate without satisfactorily completing a piece of research.

The family practice discipline in some countries have followed lead: For example, in Croatia a research project is a mandatory component of the postgraduate vocational training of family practitioners. The best of the projects are published in medical journals or presented at the national family practice conferences.

What do we research in family practice?
The subjects of research

This has become characterized by process rather than content. We have become the experts in researching processes such as:

- ➢ Communication skills
- ➢ Patient satisfaction; and
- ➢ Health services research, etc.

As can be seen in one analysis of the content of a sample of family practice research this is not to denigrate process research. Yet, the low output of clinical research is surprising. This dominates the subject matter of other medical disciplines, but is overshadowed in family practice by health services research. Of course health services research is important. However there may be a danger in some countries of family practice research being seen as mainly process research. We need to ask firstly if this is important, and then reasons for this state of affairs.

Clinical research for family practice is not as easily defined, or contained, as for other medical disciplines. Family practice clinical research can be "translation" research determining if the outcomes of specialist research are both effective and efficient in the family practice setting. But this is only one dimension of the necessary family questions of pertinence to the unique milieu of family practice.

Why has family practice research moved to process (health services) research rather than (clinical) research? Clinical research can be defined as research that attempts to inform clinical practice. It might be molecular, bench-top, based on patient contact, or epidemiological (populationbased) and still qualify. Conversely, any research of these characteristics might not be classified as clinical research. The question demands an analysis of more basic fundamentals concerning the discipline of family practice itself. Are we a process-based rather than a content based discipline, (as many, both inside and outside the discipline, assert? If not content-based, what then characterizes us? This is being addressed elsewhere. However the nub of the question revolves around the fact that for almost every disease there is a specialist. If the world is seen as in terms of diseases, then there will be a specialist to be its expert. Moreover when a student researches a disease they may find themselves becoming a specialist in the relevant discipline. Many public health specialists for example have arrived at that destination from family practice. Nevertheless it important that we are known for the illnesses and diseases were are experts in managing.

Research in family practice: the process of research

Most family practice uses descriptive techniques, many surveys, (investigating practitioners self-reported behaviours, attitudes and opinions about a range of topics). This has been so overdone that, (in some countries at least), there is good evidence of 'over-surveying', with poor responses rates and concomitant response biases as a consequence. Moreover several primary care journal editors have resolved to decline survey research as a first. What should family practice research training consist of? There is the training necessary to successfully undertake a research project (research techniques), and the ancillary, indirect, skills necessary to become an effective researcher. Research techniques Research methods Training in research methods should lead to suitable approaches taken to answer a research question. Additionally, this training would ensure that irrespective of the type of research question being asked, a quality project is undertaken. Some understanding in this is also needed for users of research to make sense of the research they read.

Bio-statistics

This is necessary for understanding the results and implications of published studies, and to be able to analyze and interpret the results of their own research activities.

Qualitative methods

These are clearly important for understanding phenomena. Qualitative research is increasingly used as an adjunct to provide depth of understanding to quantitative results. It can be used to improve the design and conduct of quantitative research.

Epidemiology

There is a need for training in both descriptive (monitoring patients with chronic diseases) and clinical epidemiology in family practice. In the past, clinical epidemiology has increased understanding about the impact of the types of morbidity patterns seen in family practice eon the interpretation of diagnostic test (lower sensitivity and positive predictive value than in specialist practice, and higher specificity and negative predictive value).

Other essential ancillary attributes
Critical thinking

Training in critical thinking encourages family practitioners to question their everyday actions. It also enables the development of necessary analytical skills to derive sensible and logical conclusions from any data collected during a research project.

Project management

Much family practice research activities involve research staff, and are funded for discrete timeframes. This invokes deadlines. Project management skills training ensures that the project is successfully carried out within the allocated budget and timeframe. Additionally, often the success for a research activity lies with the abilities and attitudes of the research staff employed to carry out the day-to-day tasks. Well managed staff are more likely to be satisfied and committed to the project.

Writing skills

These are important adjuncts to research. The skills are initially required to attract research funds and then to report the outcomes.

Presentation skills

Development of skills to present results of family practice research at conferences etc is also an important component of the dissemination of research outcomes. High quality presentations increase the perceived value of the research, in addition to the esteem of the researcher/ presenter.

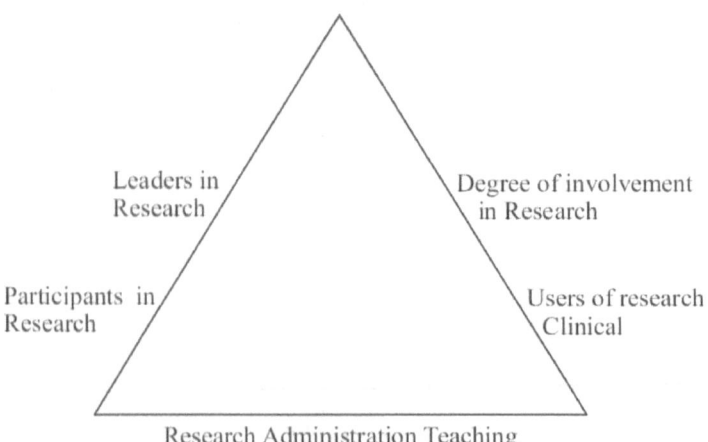

Introduction

When we look at our practice in family medicine, we are, on daily basic, involved in a huge variety of activities. We treat patients with acute diseases, reassure patients with self-limiting diseases, counsel patients with psycho-relational problems, take care problems, take care of chronic patients, prevent health problems through information and screening programs organize 24-hours continuity of care, help to identify health threats in the community, strive for equity in accessibility of health care, advocate health care for illegal residents. Family physicians are involved in a wide spectrum of interventions, where they put a lot of personal commitment and endeavour.

A critical review of the actions undertaken during one day in our family practice, will learn that some of our actions are underpinned by sound scientific evidence, quite a lot are based on "consensus", some of "common sense" and a few on "personal intuition". Looking at the literature, we will learn that a lot of pertinent questions in family medicine stay unanswered, and a lot of "scientific" evidence is not at all relevant for daily patient care in family practice. What makes research in family medicine specific? At regular intervals, the question arises why a specific research in family medicine is needed. Is it not sufficient to transpose the results of research in e.g. pediatrics, internal medicine, geriatrics to family medicine.

The fundamental answer to this question is that family medicine is a specific discipline. First of all the ecology of family is unique; the family physician in his role a first contact for all kind of health problems. deals with a huge variety of problems mostly in early stages. Symptoms are often vague, prevalence of serious diseases is low a lot of problems are self-limiting. This epidemiology makes decision making in primary care totally different from secondary care settings. Where prevalence of serious disease is much higher, illnesses are in more developed states and prognosis is often worse. This is illustrated by looking at the randomized controlled trials which are universally considered as the sources for evidence based medicine. Existing randomized controlled trials (RCTs) are very often of little use for the family physician. Most RCTs study patients with well defined diseases, inclusion and exclusion and exclusion criteria and consequently most patients in family medicine will-due to its specific epidemiology not answer to these criteria: the disease is not yet sufficiently developed, they have other concurrent health problems, and they are too old. It is very often difficult to find a study that fits the patient in front of you.

Therefore, trials in primary care are badly needed: trials that start from common complaints and symptoms, trials with few exclusion criteria, including a variety of patients comparable with the average family practice population. Diversity in the study population can be an advantage, instead of a problem. These trials should ideally be large enough since small trials tend to exaggerate intervention benefits. Yet large randomized clinical trials are not always feasible, and most of the time very costly. In primary care we will probably continue to live with the paradox that the rigor of inclusion-criteria and patient selection, needed for an RCT, is completely opposite to daily practice.

A second unique characteristic of primary care is that the context of care is very important. Non-medical factors such as the doctor-patient relationship, the cultural context, the occupational context, the support networks, the socioeconomic context, influence the diagnostic and therapeutic approach and the final outcome. There is e.g. empirical evidence that enhancing patient's expectations improves outcome.

More research on the importance of these context factors is necessary and can only be performed in the general practice setting. It is obvious that apart from "medical evidence" (evidence based medicine), we need "contextual evidence" in order to contribute to better patient care This research will evidently have to be interdisciplinary and involve other discipline such as psychology, sociology, anthropology.

A third characteristic of primary care is its strong link with and responsibility to the community. Primary care is not only directed towards individual patients, but is concerned with the community. It wants to obtain as such health gains as possible out of the limited budgets for as many community members as possible. But to achieve this, more specific research is needed: more health economic research to assess cost/benefit balances of therapeutic and diagnostic interventions and to study equity and accessibility of health care; "community diagnosis" to help uncover community related health hazards and suggest community based interventions. Results of this economic and community research can provide us with indispensable "policy evidence" to underpin social ethical decisions. More, primary care research in itself has a responsibility to the (investing society): it should try to return to this society as much as possible by maximizing through its being.

Research is being perceived by most of the old generation G.Ps if the following ways:

1. It is a specialization done by researchers only.
2. It is done in specialized lab or medical colleges or university teaching hospitals.
3. It requires lot of funds.
4. It is a full time job.
5. It is almost impossible to do research while involved in the patients' care.
6. G.Ps have not been trained to do research.
7. G.Ps have no time to do research.
8. No resource/ support available to do research.
9. No knowledge of utilization of research product.
10. Being scared of doing lot of paper work.
11. No knowledge of publishing criteria.
12. No knowledge of research methodology.

Most of the G.Ps, both old and new generations do not get involved with the research activities for the following seasons:

1. No incentives
2. Busy practices
3. Lack of resources and support e.g. computer, statistician
4. Not mandatory
5. Lack of stimulation

It is the Right Time

The discipline of family medicine has finally established itself as an academic discipline after struggling for nearly half of the 20th Century. We have defined our core concepts, knowledge and skills, although debate still exists on the fine details of the content of our work. Most universities include family medicine as a core component of their medical curricula. University departments of family medicine are now common, not only in Western Europe and North America But also in Eastern Europe and Asia where it was rarely heard of ten to twenty years ago.

In our attempt to consolidate our body of knowledge, we have acquired must research expertise in studying diagnostic process, natural history of common illnesses, and the complex interaction between medical, psychological, social and behavioural factors. In bridging the gap between medical knowledge and clinical practice, we have established a track record in the search on medical intervention in the patient's context, patient-centered outcomes, the impact of the consultation; alternative models of health care; health needs of disadvantaged groups and health promotion.

It is time for the discipline to build on its research to further advance its knowledge in the practice of medicine.

The Environment is most suitable

The rapid development of many life-saving technologies over the 20th Century has ironically perpetuated sick lives more than health ones which Ernest Gruenberg calls 'the failures of success' The cure of many acute infectious diseases has resulted in a relative rise in cancerous, degenerative, functional and psychological diseases. This is compounded with increasing health care cost and inequality in access to care (especially high-tech secondary and tertiary treatments). There are many new challenges to clinical care, health services delivery and professional development in the 21st Century. The need for quality primary care to improve health outcomes is becoming more and more apparent. As Mant et al have pointed out; research in the primary care setting is needed to provide evidence for the improvement of primary care services to patients because results from traditional research in the hospital environment are often not applicable in this context.

An audit on anticoagulant treatment for patients with atrial fibrillation in our Unit found that the use of Warfarin was not feasible in the primary car setting and only two out of 17 'eligible' patients could successfully be put on aspirin. Hospital-based management guidelines are often not applicable to primary care because out patients are different from those used in trials. Positive predictive values of diagnostic tests found in the hospital setting drop markedly in the primary care setting because of a change in diseases prevalence.

Stakeholders Seem Supportive

The WHO declared that primary health was the key to 'health for all of the year 2000' at the Al Conference on Primary Health Care in 1987, but unfortunately the role of the family doctor was not clarified. In the joint WHO-WONCA Conference in 1994 the WHO formally endorsed the contribution of family medicine to medical practice and education. Access to comprehensive, essential, quality health care was reaffirmed to be an indicator of 'Health for all in the 21st Century at the World Health Assembly in 1998. Family medicine must not miss this second opportunity to show how it can contribute to quality primary care with research evidence.

More and more governments are supporting training in family medicine for doctors working in primary care. The development has been rapid in Asia can Central Europe in the last two decades. Family medicine was almost non-existent before 1986 in China, but in 1997 the Chinese Government made in a policy to promote family medicine training for primary care doctors. In Lithuania, Latvia and Estonia the number of family doctors increased from tens in the nineties to thousands providing primary health care for 50 to 80% of their populations in 2003 [personal communication from Prof Leona Vanus, 2003. In Hong Kong, the number of family medicine training posts has increased by more than 10 times from 20 in 1993 to 346 in 2002].

Our discipline has the largest number of members, ranging from 10% in Asian countries to 70% in the Netherlands, who have some academic links through their involvements in vocational training and undergraduate teaching. [Personal communication from Professors Chris Van Weel, Lee-GanGoh, Zorayda E Leopando, Yuan Gu and RyukiKassai], although we do not have as many full time academia as other disciplines.

These family doctors can greatly expand the research capacity of family medicine if they are motivated and supported to do so through networking with academic departments and each other. Research funding bodies are starting to see the importance and relevance of investing in primary care and health services research, which provide great opportunities for family medicine. More and more clinical trials include patients from primary care and require the participation from family doctors.

Research is by most family practitioners seen as a specialist endeavour or a task necessary to be undertaken by the few family practitioners, who wants to become academics. Research is not felt or understood to be an integrated part of good primary patient care, which should be carried out by all family practitioners. This lack of understanding of research as an integral part of both intellectual and practical family medicine is a big problem for the profession. It greatly influences the thinking and the attitude of those people, who determine and administer the working content and the conditions in primary care the politicians, practice managers, health economists and other primary care administrators.

Research themes in Family Medicine

What are the important questions in family medicine? This depends on the "eyes that see", but it is more likely that a curious family doctor can formulate interesting research questions and find research methods which are applicable to primary care, than a doctor who has no experience in family medicine.

There are many relevant clinical questions to be answered. Some patients are only seen by the family doctor, who both diagnose and managing the patient's health problem, without referring to other physicians. Some of these problems can be answered by using clinical controlled trials, but sometimes these methods are not practical in a primary care setting, and other methods have to be used or even developed. Some of the problems encountered in family practice are related to patients with vague symptoms from many parts of the body. The biomedical approach to understand these patients are insufficient, and research methods from other sciences have to be applied. A significant portion of the research in primary care should focus on health problems most of the people have most of the time (Nutting 1994).

Epidemiological studies are important since they form the basis for our knowledge of primary care. The epidemiological research requires data about patient's disease episodes from their beginning as unspecified symptoms to a defined pathological entity, which can be labeled with a diagnostic term. In order to do this and compare results internationally, a comprehensive classification of patients' reason for encounter, process of care and the family doctor's diagnostic terminology is necessary.

Health care services research is another important topic family doctors should be involved in Teamwork and co-operation between the different health care workers and between the different levels of health care is core issues for a well functioning health care system and for the optimal use of resources. The way we deliver healthcare to people has a great impact on their health but also on recruitment and sustainability of healthcare personnel. This is especially true in rural and remote areas. We need to know more about the impact of organizing the health services has both on patient's health seeking behaviour and on the use of resources.

In some societies where changes in organization and financing of health care services changes all the time, there is a need for monitoring and documenting the effect of such changes. Although the changes are mainly administrative, they have a large impact of the family doctors working conditions and the delivery of health care to people. Other themes are prevention of major health problems, especially those related to lifestyle behaviour like smoking, excessive drinking, eating and lack of physical exercise. Prevention of infectious diseases such as measles, AIDS and malaria and early detection of treatable cancer diseases such as cervical and breast cancer is another large area for primary care research. Disease mongering has become a real threat to the balance in healthcare.

Strong pharmaceutical and medical industries, special interest groups among patients, politicians influence the demand for care by the general public. This can change the patient's reason for encounter, and influence the family practitioners work away from detecting and treating patients with specific diseases towards dealing with resourceful and demanding patients, whose main concern is fear of disease, but with no sign or symptom of such.

In a world where individualism and money play an increasing role, we as family doctors have to look for solidarity and fairness in the distribution of the health care resources. These are just some of many research themes relevant for family practitioners. Methodology In order to carry out research in a primary care setting, special methodology and research design apply. These have to be developed and described by the family doctors themselves together with other professionals working in primary care. WONCA support this development through its support of the WONCA International Classification Committee (WICC) and other WORKING PARTIES AND GROUPS. WICC has through the years been one of WONCA'S most productive committees. Its main task has been to develop a number of comprehensive classification for primary care – the best known being the International Classification for Primary Care, now available in its second edition (ICPC-2) (WICC 1998) and in an electronic format ICPC-2-E (Okkes 2000). This classification must be able to communicate with classifications used in other levels of the health service. Great effort is therefore done to ensure a good mapping between ICD-10 and ICPC-2. ICD-10 can be mapped to other major classifications like SNOMED-CT-10-CM, ICD-10-AM, and this ensures that there is a conversion between these classifications and ICPC 2.

The fruitful relationship between WONCA and the WHO has resulted in the establishment of a working group between the Centre Heads of the WHO Collaborating Centres of Classifications and WICC. The task is to see whether WHO can adopt ICPC-2 AS member of the family of classifications. Icpc-2 is missing link and should be the physician's reason for encounter. Another tool which WICC has developed, in order to facilitate international communication and understanding of concepts related to family medicine, is the "Wonca Dictionary of General/Family Practice". This dictionary is now in print, and it is the first attempt to have a comprehensive source for understanding the words and the terms we use to describe many of the important concepts in family practice. It is based on "An international glossary for general family practice" which contained mostly scientific terms related to family practice. Other tools have been adapted to the specific needs in family practice; among these are the DUSOI/WONCA severity of illness charts and the COOP/WONCA functional assessment charts. They have both been extensively tested internationally in family practice and have shown to be useful and valid for specific research purposes. In order to gain wider use, they need to be developed further and tested in primary care settings in different parts of the world. Other health outcome measures have been developed and modified for use in primary and ambulatory care and should be available to family practitioners throughout the world. Practice activity recording methods and software programmes, which can retrieve data from the electronic patient records, are examples of other tools, which can help and promote research in family practice.

In order to answer research questions about patients with many and/or vague somatic symptoms, health problems which do not represent defined clinical entitles, or understand why patients behave in a strange way, we have to look for "new" research methods. To gain insight into these kinds of problems, qualitative research methods are needed, and these methods are relatively new to medicine. They are not yet integrated and approved by the dominant scientific bodies in most medical schools. These methods have to be learned from subjects like anthropology, psychology and sociology, and include interview, focus groups observation and other methods, which can help us to understand our patients. These methods must be developed further by family practitioners to fit the research needs of family medicine.

FOR FURTHER READING

1. Schildmann J, Cushing A, Doyal L, et al; Breaking bad news: experiences, views and difficulties of preregistration house officers. Palliat Med. 2005 Mar;19(2):93-8. [abstract]
2. Farrell, M.; Breaking Bad news. In Shaw, T. and Sanders, K. (Eds.) Foundation of Nursing Studies Dissemination Series. Vol. 1.No. 2.2002
3. Barnett MM; Effect of breaking bad news on patients' perceptions of doctors. J R Soc Med. 2002 Jul;95(7):343-7. [abstract]
4. Simpson C; When hope makes us vulnerable: a discussion of patient-healthcare provider interactions in the context of hope. Bioethics. 2004 Sep; 18(5):428-47. [abstract]
5. Mental Capacity Act 2005; Office of Public Sector Information Public Acts 2005
6. VandeKieft GK; Breaking bad news. Am Fam Physician. 2001 Dec 15;64(12): 1975-8. [abstract]
7. Dias L, Chabner BA, Lynch TJ Jr, et al; Breaking bad news: a patient's perspective. Oncologist. 2003;8(6):587-96. [abstract].
8. Breaking Bad News; Breakindbadnews.com; *Useful resources for UK Health Professionals.*
9. Breaking Bad News Regional Guidelnes; National Council For Hospice And Specialist Palliative Care Services 2002.
10. Brod T.M., Cohen M.M., Weinstock E. (1986) *Cancer disclosure: communicating the diagnosis to patients – a videotape.* Medcom, Inc. Garden GroveCA. Buckman R. (1994) *How to break bad news: a guide for health care professionals.* Papermac, London.
11. Christensen P. J. & Kenney J. N. (1990) *Nursing Process Application of Conceptual Models.* St. Louis Mosby.
12. Cushing A.M., Jones A. (1995) *Evaluation of a breaking bad news course for medical students.* Medic al Education. 29:430-35.

13. Henslin J.M. (1995), *Sociology: A down-to-earth approach.* Boston: Allyn and Bacon.

14. Maguire P., Faulkner A. (1988) *Improve the counselling skills of doctors and nurses in cancer care* BMJ 297, 847-849.

15. Sanson Fisher (1992) *How to break bad news to cancer patients.* An interactional skills manual for interns. The Professional Education and Training Committee of the New South Wales Cancer Council and the Postgraduate Medical Council of NSW Australia, Kings Cross, NSW Australia.

16. Baile, Walter F. et al, "SPIRES – a six step protocol for delivering bad news: application to the patient with cancer. The Oncologist 5.4 (2000), 302-34.

17. Modified from Smilkstein G: The family APGAR: A proposal for family function test and its use by physicians, J. Family Practice 6(6), 1978. Reprinted by permission of Appleton and Lange, Inc.

18. Brod et al, 1986; Maguire and Faulkner, 1988; Sanson-Fisher, 1992, Buckman, 1994; Cushing and Jones 1995). From Silverman J., Kurtz S.M., Draper J. (1998) Skills for Communicating with Patients. Radcliffe Medical Press Oxford.